KEEPING BALANCE

A psychologist's experience of chronic illness and disability

Katherine Cuthbert

Matador
5 Weir Road
Kibworth Beauchamp
Leicester LE8 0LQ, UK
Tel: (+44) 116 279 2299
Fax: (+44) 116 279 2277
Email: books@troubador.co.uk
Web: www.troubador.co.uk/matador

ISBN 978 1848762 091

British Library Cataloguing in Publication Data.
A catalogue record for this book is available from the British Library.

Typeset in 11.5pt Book Antiqua by Troubador Publishing Ltd, Leicester, UK
Printed and bound by TJ International Ltd, Padstow, Cornwall, UK

Matador is an imprint of Troubador Publishing Ltd

For Pete
With love and thanks - for everything

also
In loving memory of a very special friend
Mary Elizabeth Hallows
18th June 1951 to 28th May 2009

My thanks are given to Mary in the acknowledgements section of this book
and something of her story is told in later pages.

And in admiration of those many people who live well with more severe
illness and greater disability than I have experienced

Contents

Acknowledgements

I want to thank the friends who have read the manuscript of this book at various stages during its completion. I am especially grateful to Nerys Hughes and Marion Polihroniadis who I feel have been with me on the journey.

From very early on Nerys has reacted to my writing almost on a chapter by chapter basis. She has provided thoughtful written reaction - both supportive and helpfully critical – and we have talked together regularly about how things were going. It has been tremendously motivating to have someone who was prepared to take such a close interest and give the time to react and comment in this way.

I think that Marion was the first person (apart from Pete) whom I told about the project so her early enthusiasm was important. Marion is a fellow psychologist. We have had many discussions which have combined the personal and the psychological in ways that have been tremendously helpful. Marion commented on and reacted to an early set of draft chapters and then a later more complete draft during weekend visits to each other.

Two ex-colleagues also reacted helpfully to drafts at varying levels of completion. Marilyn Hackney, who taught psychology with me for a number of years, read an early incomplete draft. Professor Gaye Heathcote, a sociologist, and my head of department for a number of years, gave me positive early encouragement and then read the almost final manuscript when she had more time after retirement.

I have had help from my very good friends Martin and Mary Hallows. They support each other in the joint challenge of both having MS. They read the draft manuscript and gave me their approval. It was important to me to have this reaction from others in the same situation as myself.

A number of friends have read parts of the manuscript – most especially the outline, preface and chapter summaries – and then provided reactions. Others have inquired regularly about progress. Having people interested in an ongoing writing project of this kind has been most important and I thank you all.

More recently some newer friends, Ann Macaulay, Audrey Pierpoint, Jean Steel, Mary King, Norma Dunbar, Pat Cairns and Pat Warrener have given me much appreciated encouragement. They are recent members of the Life Writing Group within our local U3A. We have enjoyed sharing with each other experiences from our lives.

Within my family, I am pleased that my parents, Ieuan and Frances John, were able to read parts of an early draft of my manuscript. I want to thank my sisters, Mair Lustig and Ceridwen John, for their reading contribution and for their continuing support and encouragement.

Most especially, I wish to record my thanks to my husband Pete. When someone becomes disabled not only is the person's own life changed irrevocably, but so is that of their nearest and dearest. Pete has given me the greatest support and continuing love since the time of my diagnosis in 1993.

In relation to this particular project he has read and commented on quite a few drafts, helped in re-orientation when things were not working out, and rescued me from many word-processing difficulties. In addition, among other things, he has been chief bike mechanic and puncture repairer. Most of all he has helped me to stay sane and positive when times have been especially difficult.

Acknowledgements

Finally, I would like to give some thanks in relation to professional advice and support received. Under the auspices of the Literary Consultancy helpfully critical feedback was provided in relation to an early draft of my manuscript. More recently, as part of the Matador process, the full manuscript has been very well edited to provide that final 'polish'. My thanks to everybody at Matador for organising the production and publishing of my book.

Acknowledgements

Preface

Why have I decided to write about my life? Previously this possibility would just not have entered into my consciousness. My life has been an ordinary one. I am not famous. I have not led an exciting or remarkable life. But in the summer of 1993 everything changed, suddenly and drastically. I was diagnosed with multiple sclerosis. I had entered a new world in which illness and disability would be continuing parts of my experience.

This new world was different and strange, but it is one which considerable numbers of people find themselves forced to enter – without any freedom to refuse. Inevitably, many original landmarks disappear. We need to find our way through a different kind of existence – physically, emotionally and psychologically.

My most important reason for writing this book, as indicated by its sub-title, is because I am a psychologist. I have found that my knowledge and understanding as a psychologist has helped me in the processes of adjusting to, and managing life with chronic illness and disability. My central theme is that psychological understanding makes a contribution to practical adjustment. This psychological content is not presented formally, or in an academic way. I tell the 'story' of my psychological adjustment alongside the various other aspects of my ongoing experience of life, including my efforts to keep cycling and the building of our new house.

My second reason has, in some ways, a more selfish foundation, but I hope with wider benefits. As a person newly diagnosed with MS, I began to keep a diary. I have found, as with academic writing, that the process and discipline of writing helped me to clarify my thoughts. New ideas, and new understandings of my experience emerged as I reflected on what was happening to me, and attempted to write about it. The discipline of writing for possible publication prompted me to extend both reflection and exploration. As a consequence, my writing has certainly been of personal benefit. I hope that this reflection and the consequent changes in the way that I live my life will be of relevance to others.

But who are these others? For whom have I written the book? Probably, many readers will be those who are like myself to a greater or lesser extent - people who have developed a chronic illness. Many, but by no means all of those who have a chronic illness will also be disabled to some degree. Others will have become disabled primarily through injury and might well not consider themselves to be ill. But the members of this combined group will have the common experience that they have become ill and/or disabled. Those who have been disabled from birth might find some aspects of interest, but will probably feel, justifiably, that the book is not primarily addressed to them and, in many ways, cannot encompass their experience.

But can a book like this 'encompass' anybodys experience? I do not think so. This book provides an offering of ideas - filtered through my experience, and knowledge of psychology. Those of us who become disabled come to disability from all sorts of prior lives. Our different, unique lives influence how we cope, and what might be relevant and useful to us. We are not *the* disabled – we are people with all sorts and varieties of experience, qualities and capabilities.

Hopefully, some psychologists and students of psychology will read this book. It should be of particular interest to sub-groups within the profession such as health psychologists and clinical and counselling psychologists. Quite clearly this cannot be a 'textbook' examination of the relevant issues. There is little discussion of research evidence. There is bound to be a degree of simplification. But the book, by its nature, involves something of an 'inside' examination of the experience of coping with disability. Thus, it has the added value of providing a useful complement to the necessarily 'outside' perspective of non-disabled psychologists.

But what if you are neither disabled, nor a student of psychology? Why should this book be of interest to you - the 'ordinary' reader? There are a couple of related reasons. Firstly, most of us experience problems of one kind or another during our lives. Reading how others have coped, even with quite different kinds of life challenges, is likely to be of benefit. Secondly, we will all grow old. Although the current tendency is to emphasise the more beneficial aspects of this life stage, the chance of experiencing illness and incapacity increases. Coping with disability is not an easy matter at any stage in life, but those who have lived a long time with disability will likely have developed the knowledge and skills for coping positively in these circumstances. People with disabilities can often be stigmatised, but our experience can support the achievement of successful coping.

Since this book is a memoir of my life, inevitably it has a personal focus. I hope, though, that I can convey something, in more general terms, of what it is like to be chronically ill and disabled. Since becoming disabled myself, I have been hugely impressed by the ability of many disabled people to cope positively. Psychologists also are beginning to become interested in the demonstrated ability to manage well shown by many in these circumstances.

This is quite a complex narrative, and I have chosen not to write in wholly sequential terms, though there is some time sequence involved through the chapters. The first few chapters review my life before MS so providing a context for my later coping, but through most of the book there is a greater emphasis on the various activities and experiences that contribute to my life. This may make for some discontinuity here and there – hopefully forgivable. Any life and the ongoing adaptation that it involves, is complex and dynamic and is not necessarily best depicted in strictly sequential terms.

It might be you do not wish to read the book in a wholly sequential manner. Non-psychologists might find that the psychological content of one or two chapters is too dominant and possibly a bit 'heavy' and that my own story becomes less central in these discussions. This probably happens in chapter two especially and since it comes so near to the beginning, non-psychologists may wish to skip over it. Later chapters will still make sense without it.

On the other hand, much of chapter two is about matters of self and identity. A concern with self and the personal question of 'Who am I?' is something that, in the post-modern world, most of us will feel at least some pressure to address. Those of us forced to confront the changes posed by the onset of disability may have more need than others to confront this question.

This book has been written over a lengthy period. I first started jotting down notes on my encounter with MS at the end of 1994. I gradually developed a parallel list of psychological ideas that seemed helpful in my new situation. At that stage I was primarily exploring my experience for myself.

Gradually these notes and my diary record evolved and provided the basis for this more integrated commentary. The extended development does mean that I wrote some of the chapters quite a while prior to publication. Some have been revised as events or experience changed but where it seemed more important to preserve the immediacy of my reactions at the time, no revision has been attempted. Thus, in various ways, this is an account of my journey through illness and disability, partly as it happened, but also with some retrospective reflection.

A final important point is addressed primarily to any academic psychologists who might read this book. This account of my life is certainly not a textbook, but it does make use of and draw upon the writings of other psychologists and other relevant commentators. Most readers will not be academics and exhaustive referencing is not possible or altogether appropriate. I hope that I have done sufficient to allow interested readers to follow up references if they so wish and to indicate to academic readers the general nature of my sources.

Chapter One

Diagnosis and Before

It was July 29th 1993 and we were approaching the end of a cycling holiday in Bavaria. With my husband Pete, I had arrived in Berchtesgarten the previous afternoon having cycled the twenty odd miles from our last overnight stay at the town of Inzell. It had been another beautiful ride, now with the mountains all around us, but still the cycling was not too strenuous.

We were on a fairly leisurely ten day touring holiday through a corner of Bavaria. The tour involved cycling one day, then staying two nights in a traditional Bavarian *Gasthaus*. On the second day we could take a further cycle day trip, or walk, or just potter around in a more lazy way. The cycling tour was organised to the degree that hotels were booked, route maps provided, and luggage transported from hotel to hotel. It was an easy way of having a touring holiday without too much preliminary effort.

On this particular non-cycling day, we had just walked down into the valley from our hotel higher up in the town in order to visit a local salt mine. We had walked a little through the tunnels, ridden on a narrow gauge electric powered train, and slid down to lower levels on a polished wooden 'slide'. It had been great fun but certainly nothing very strenuous. Strangely though I found that my left leg was 'giving way' a little as I walked – not completely, so there was no dramatic collapse but enough to let me know that something was not quite right.

Later that day, as I climbed the stairs to our hotel room, my leg felt heavy. It was a real effort to get up the two flights.

The next day we moved on to the final stop of our holiday. This involved a cycle ride of around 25 miles. Fortunately my legs seemed to be working better on the bike than off it. It was a beautiful ride, moving slowly away from the high mountains, and then, in the afternoon, cycling alongside the wide and turbulent Salzach river. The latter part of our ride was on the riverside cycle path through the city of Salzburg. Then onwards a few final miles to the village and hotel where we were staying for the night.

The following day was free to explore Salzburg. By this time I was feeling quite concerned that my legs were not altogether functioning normally. We took the train in rather than cycling again, and took advantage of available transport around the city instead of walking, as we would normally have done. I didn't feel that I was capable of walking too far.

On the final day of our holiday walking the half mile or so from the hotel to the station for the beginning of our journey home was difficult, with a degree of numbness in my feet combined with a feeling that was something like 'pins and needles'. My legs were certainly not operating in the smooth and easy way one normally takes completely for granted. I was getting worried about what was going on.

These various symptoms obviously indicated some kind of serious problem so as soon as we were home I booked a visit to my GP. He was somewhat dismissive – or reassuring – depending on your view. He thought that my problems resulted from the cycling I had done during the holiday. I wasn't convinced. The cycling hadn't been that strenuous. I wasn't super fit, but reasonably so. I had cycled more extensively in the past without anything like this happening. After a couple more visits and no sign of any improvement he organised an appointment with the neurology registrar at the nearest hospital on August 19th.

The registrar listened to my account of my symptoms and conducted some of the initial standard tests to check neurological responses. He checked the sensation in my legs; scratched along the underside of my foot with a sharp instrument; asked me to stand up with eyes closed while he was ready to catch me if I lost balance; and got me to stretch out an arm and then bring it back to touch my nose, again with my eyes closed. There were probably a few other little challenges I have forgotten. Certainly he was taking things seriously and wanted to admit me into the neurological ward at the hospital, after I had collected the necessaries for an immediate overnight stay. I had suspected that there was something important amiss, but this degree of urgency was still unexpected and rather disturbing.

I was in hospital for three days. For quite a bit of the time I was just sitting around but there were a few further tests. The one that made the greatest impression was being 'wired up' with scalp EEG (electroencephalograph) recorders and then having to watch rapidly changing geometric figures on a screen. Doctors were not that available or communicative but I managed to get some information from a young assistant doctor. It seemed that the most likely possibilities were either a brain tumour or multiple sclerosis. I had thought that the latter was a possibility so it wasn't a total shock – but it was still seriously worrying to have a medic suggesting this as a probability.

Compared with many people's experience of an MS diagnosis mine was pretty fast. This has some benefits – you know the worst quickly. But the sudden transition from being reasonably fit and, as far as I knew quite healthy, to finding that I had a serious chronic illness made for something of a disruption to normal equilibrium. At this point the diagnosis was still unofficial and uncertain.

The final step in the diagnosis process was an MRI (magnetic resonance imaging) brain and spinal cord scan on the morning of August 26th. Most will have seen a film of this process happening – either in a medical documentary, or during a hospital 'soap'. You lie on your back on a waist high platform, head immobilised. The platform then slides backwards into the relatively small opening of the long, white, tube-like apparatus, all taking around 20 to 30 minutes. In itself the process was not too disturbing, but of course, I had concerns about the outcome. We would obviously have to wait a little while for the results.

Meanwhile, back in the usual world, despite our departure from ordinary existence, life was, of course, carrying on as normal. It was the August bank holiday weekend. We decided on some essential escape from our sudden immersion in hospitals and looming illness and booked ourselves into a hotel in Durham – a place we had never visited before. So, with a weekend away, we looked forward to some degree of normality.

The hotel, a more expensive choice perhaps than in more usual circumstances, was fantastic in quite a number of ways, and close to the old city centre. We made good use of a superb swimming pool, which looked out over the river. At least I could still swim, even if a little less energetically than usual! We had an attractive bedroom and took advantage of the room service provision of breakfast in bed.

We were able to get out and about, though my walking capability was not too good. My legs weren't working well and the feeling of heaviness was persisting. We discovered the hotel had a loan wheelchair available, though the idea of actually using one was quite horrifying in many ways. Only a few weeks previously I had walked six or seven miles – apparently without any problem – on one of the non-cycling days of our holiday. But for this weekend, if we could do more things and get to more places by using a wheelchair then it was worth it.

A busy few days followed – an excellent antidote to the stress of the hospital experience. With Durham explored, especially the old city and the Cathedral and the river – we wheelchaired along the banks, and took a rowing boat out onto the river. We also made a few trips into the surrounding countryside.

In addition there was some space and time to talk, and think, and begin to assess what was happening. I was very lucky that as soon as the likely seriousness of my symptoms became apparent, Pete was hugely supportive and took the attitude that it was *our* problem, with which we would cope together, rather than just *my* illness.

Clearly, life was going to change, though we could not tell at that stage by how much. So, how had we...I...got to where we were? What sort of life were we leading? On what kind of resources and past experience were we, and I able to draw? There would be adaptations needed for both of us and I was very fortunate to be able to feel that Pete would give me every support that was possible. But, given that I was the one who had succumbed to this disease, I soon began to realise that even with the most supportive partner, I would be on the coping and adjustment front line. So, while this story of living with MS is ours, it still has to be primarily mine.

What was life like before July 1993? What kind of family did I come from? Would my childhood and later experiences provide the foundation on which to cope with the current challenge?

I was brought up in the small Welsh university and seaside town of Aberystwyth, positioned at the mid-point on the sweep of Bae Ceredigion. I wasn't actually born there, but in a small terraced cottage in Tonypandy, in the Rhondda valley, the home of my maternal grandparents. My parents (Ieuan Gwilym John and Frances Rose John) were both from the South Wales valleys and from mining 'stock'. They went to the same secondary school, then they met each other again in London, just before the war, where my father was a post-graduate research student at The London School of Economics, and my mother was a teacher. They had made that challenging journey from a working class background, through higher education and into professional life in the difficult period of the mid nineteen thirties.

My parents were married towards the close of the war – on February

10th 1945. When my father was finally discharged from his war service in the navy he secured a lecturing post in the Department of International Politics at the University College of Wales at Aberystwyth. I was born on November 14th 1946 and was brought by my mother to join my father in Aberystwyth when I was a few weeks old.

So, I grew up through the nineteen fifties and early sixties in a middle class home, but where, in common with most people in the middle years of the last century, there was not too much money around. We acquired a car when I was eleven, and a television a few years later, although my mother had very sensibly bought a washing machine rather sooner. I don't know when knitting machines became readily available, but my mother must have bought one quite early on. One of my abiding childhood memories is of hearing its back and forth, 'clickety-clack' movement as my mother knitted something for one or other of us children.

I was the eldest child, my younger twin sisters were born in 1949. I was named Katherine after my grandmother, but my sisters both had Welsh names – Ceridwen (usually shortened to Ceri) and Mair. Being the eldest, with twins as younger sisters did have disadvantages. I was expected to take some extra responsibilities, and the two of them could, on occasion, 'gang up' against me. But we got on together reasonably well – most of the time.

Looking back, Aberystwyth was a good place in which to grow up. I had an easy, comfortable and happy childhood with no major traumas. Although obviously less provided with material goods, it was a childhood which was in many ways freer, and less constrained than is usual for children today. We lived in a three-storied terraced house, not too far from the railway station and the shops, and opposite to one of the two Church of England Parish churches. (As a Welsh town Aberystwyth has a preponderance of chapels.)

We played out in the streets – there weren't too many cars around.

There were also interesting places immediately nearby that we could get to without any parental supervision. Down the end of the road was Cae Sienkin (Jenkin's field). This was actually the land around (or below) the university chemistry laboratories which were situated at the top of the hill. The grounds were not kept as neat as they would be today.

The area provided the kids of the street with a useful, informal adventure playground. There was a stand of pine trees on one side. One tree in particular was just right for swinging and climbing on. I was quite proud that I could get right to the top and it was a place of seclusion for when my sisters were aggravating me, or life was feeling otherwise difficult in some way. I could be sitting up at the top of the tree and nobody would know that I was there. On the other side of the route up to the labs there was a rather jungly growth of bushes and shrubs, some of which were suitable for secret dens and associated games.

Living in a seaside town meant that we could easily get to the local beach, although not initially on our own. There was then no public swimming pool in Aberystwyth, but we were very lucky to have some access to the university baths. As far as I remember I started going to the pool when I was tall enough to stand in the shallow end with my head above water. My father used to take us swimming on a Saturday morning, and after school on a Wednesday afternoon, or early evening.

I can't actually remember learning to swim, but I became proficient fairly quickly. It was the only school sport in which I participated with any degree of enthusiasm. (I wasn't much good at the usual kind of organised competitive games which involved manipulating a ball in some way.) During the summer, we also swam in the sea. We would go down after school. The part where we all swam was pebbly (as was most of Aberystwyth beach), steeply shelving, and with breakwaters for jumping and diving from – a good swimming beach.

In addition to swimming Aberystwyth offered good opportunities for walking immediately around the town. My parents were both keen walkers and so we joined in the outings early on. You could have some good walks straight from our house – down along the river Rheidol; through the woods, around the golf links and then back down to the promenade; up Constitution hill and then along the cliff path to the next bay; or down to the harbour, across the river Ystwyth and along the beach in the opposite direction. I absorbed the beauty of this environment, but in a rather taken for granted kind of way.

When we had acquired a car outings further afield were easier. The first serious mountain I climbed was Cader Idris – about twenty five miles north of Aberystwyth and south of Barmouth and the Mawddach estuary. We would take the path from the Tal-y-Llyn (lake) side. The very first part of the approach is flat, through open woodland, but then, very soon, you are climbing steeply alongside a rushing stream with pools and waterfalls. Then the gradient eases off and the landscape becomes more open – you really feel up in the mountains. The next stage of the climb is around the side of the cwm. The waters of Llyn Cau are contained within this, and precipitous and dramatic cliffs tower above the lake. The gradient lessens somewhat for the final approach to the top. I can still remember the great sense of achievement at reaching the summit; and if the weather is good the views are spectacular.

The other physical activity I enjoyed was roller-skating. There was a time in my childhood when I think that I roller-skated wherever I could. There was some good roller-skating territory near to home. There was one wide, smooth pavement area a street away. Also, more extensively, there was Plas Crug which is a tree lined avenue, without cars but with three tarmacked 'lanes'. This was just down the road and round the corner from our house. Another slightly more reckless bit of roller-skating that we enjoyed was effortless skating down the road of a nearby hill. We squatted down on our heels and then zig-zagged down. Probably we stationed someone at the bottom to check for cars!

In addition I roller-skated the Saturday shopping errands I did for my grandparents who lived just round the corner from our house.

If this account of an active, outdoor childhood gives the impression that I was a bit of a tomboy, it is correct – I saw myself that way. I didn't like dolls and had no desire to play with them. I didn't think that they were interesting. All the dolls in the house ended up with one of my sisters regardless of who got them in the first instance. Apparently, when I was three my parents gave me a doll's pram as a birthday present. I was upset at this. What I had really wanted was a tricycle like the one owned by a boy a couple of doors away!

Most detailed memories, and certainly the development of opinions about the education I was receiving, come from my time at the local grammar school. In 1958 it was either the grammar school if you passed the 11+ or the secondary modern if you didn't.

We walked to school, calling for friends along the way, around three-quarters of a mile. Our way was up and over a steep hill, and then across one of the main roads into town, a journey we did four times every day. We did what I don't think any children would do now – we came home at lunch time for a cooked meal. My father also walked home from his university room in the old college on the promenade at the other end of town. Having left her teaching job at the end of the war, my mother's 'job', as was more typical in the 1950s, was looking after home and family.

I can still easily remember those lunch time meals. One favourite for me was shepherd's pie made from the final remains of the weekend roast. On the other hand stuffed hearts were not top of my list since there were always some tough and gristly bits. There was always a pudding too – treacle tart, or a steamed sponge were ones to especially look forward to. My mother, to some degree, had to cook two different meals. My father, unusually for those times, has been a lifelong vegetarian because his parents made that moral commitment.

Ardwyn Grammar School was a medium sized fairly traditional co-educational grammar school, as probably most were back in 1958. The teachers still wore gowns to lessons. We girls had to keep our school hats on as we walked home and through the town.

There were some distinguishing features. This was a *Welsh* grammar school and Welsh was the first language for around half of the pupils. In the first two forms pupils were 'streamed' not according to ability, but according to whether or not they spoke Welsh. The Welsh speakers learned through the medium of Welsh. (Now, there are separate English and Welsh comprehensive schools.) From the third form we were divided into science and arts streams. We were mixed up in terms of language and mostly taught through the medium of English. Those of us who had started in the English stream continued to learn Welsh, but it was Welsh taught as though it was a foreign language!

I was a reasonably enthusiastic pupil, but in common with most school children, I wasn't wholly satisfied with the teaching I received. I felt particularly critical over the teaching of Welsh. Welsh was being used all around us – by other pupils, in assembly and in the cultural activities of the school. Outside school, it was spoken in the community and on the radio. Yet we still learned Welsh through the same grammar based, and largely written approach taken for languages such as French or German. As a consequence I still could not speak Welsh fluently by the time I had completed an O level in the subject. It seemed such a waste of a great deal of time. I had no objections to learning Welsh – I just would have liked to be able to speak it!

Another frustration related to the requirement to specialise, at the end of our second year, in either arts or science subjects. I knew I wanted to take the science route, but I also enjoyed history and would have liked to continue this subject. I found it annoying this was impossible and felt critical of the necessity for us to specialise so early on.

One part of our grammar school curriculum which was unusual, and of which I whole heartedly approved, was a 'lesson' called Debate. We had debate sessions from the first form upwards right through to the sixth. They took up one lesson period every week. There was a considerable degree of pupil 'power' allowed in this context. One of us chaired each debate session, and we also chose the topics for debate. A pupil proposed the motion and presented his or her position. There was an opposing speech and seconders on each side. Then the debate was open to the rest of the class.

In my first term at the school I was elected to chair the debate sessions in my class, frustratingly because what I really wanted was to take part in the debate, rather than spending my time calling other people to speak. The topics chosen were of current political or social interest. Generally, the teacher who was taking the class would let us get on with the debate without any interference.

As I came from a family where politics and current affairs was of considerable interest, I enjoyed the opportunity to contribute to these debates. Looking back, they were also of great educational value. If you took to the business of making your case seriously, then these debates provided good experience of developing an argued position.

During my sixth form years, but obviously out of school, I was a member, and then chairperson of the local Young Socialists. We made a contribution in the Ceredigion constituency for the 1964 general election. It was quite exciting because we hoped that Labour might be able to oust the long-standing local Liberal MP. We stuffed envelopes, did some canvassing and attended a few old style rousing election meetings. We celebrated with great enthusiasm when Labour won both locally and nationally.

During my teenage years holidays with my family were an important part of the summer experience. Usually, at this time we had a camping holiday for around three weeks somewhere in Scotland. The Scottish highlands were a major favourite of my father. We returned to camp sites at Pitlochry, at Loch Morlich in the Cairngorms, and at Oban on the west coast a number of times. I got to love the beauty of the Scottish scenery also – the heather clad hills and the dark peaty rivers around Pitlochry; the pine fringed lochs, the ancient Caledonian forest, and the looming, rounded mountains of the Cairngorms; and the sea lochs with their seaweed shores and views of islands beyond on the west coast. We walked a great deal but there were also so many spots where you could just sit and absorb the beauty around you.

In the second sixth form year it was taken pretty much for granted that I would apply to university. Both my parents had been through higher education. Many of my peers were doing the same and applying either to university or teacher training college. I have no statistics for this but it seems likely the population of Aberystwyth tended towards the middle class. As well as the university, the Welsh Plant Breeding Station, the National Library of Wales, county administration and local businesses provided important sources of employment, proportionately influential in a small town. Thus, from the grammar school the percentage entry of pupils into higher education was almost certainly higher than would have generally been the case through the country in the mid nineteen sixties.

Because I had an interest in educational innovation I was particularly keen to investigate the new universities established in the early sixties. In the end I made Keele University – the oldest of the new, taking its first students in 1950 – my first choice. As a critic of early specialisation, I was enthusiastic about their first, or Foundation Year course, which provided a strong antidote to specialisation.

I arrived at Keele as a 'fresher' student at the end of September 1965. It wasn't the easiest beginning since it was a very foggy day and trains were delayed. I was stuck at Shrewsbury station for what seemed like ages. By the time I eventually arrived at the university the reception process for new students had closed down. It was a while before I could find somebody who could give me directions to find my room in one of the residential halls. After that I soon made contact with some fellow first year students and got settled in.

After an introductory week we embarked on the Foundation Year (FY) experience. A central component was the FY lecture series. There were two, hour long, lectures everyday through the academic year – at 9 o'clock and 11 o'clock. Around four hundred students filled the lecture theatre, which had been especially built for FY lectures. The lectures themselves (all 230 of them!) provided an extensive overview of important scientific, historical, political, social and philosophical ideas. It was certainly a strong antidote to my earlier A level specialisation.

The FY lecture series was not the only component of the overall FY programme. There were also termly and year long more specialised courses, but still with a 'broadening' intent. A 'sessional' course involved weekly classes through the academic year. I, like all the other students had to take a sessional course in a subject area which was different from those I had followed for A level. This was going to be my opportunity to study history – but it didn't happen. The history of modern Europe sessional I wanted to take was oversubscribed. We had to draw lots to decide who would have to leave the course. I was one of the unlucky ones!

The degree course itself followed after the completion of the foundation year. This continued the Keele tradition of requiring a bridging of the 'two cultures'. All Keele degrees were then joint honours. We had to study two principal subjects for three years. Two subsidiary subjects each taken for one year were also required. In choosing their courses, humanities or social science students had to take at least one science course. Science students had to choose at least one non science course. As my principal subjects I chose biology from the sciences, and the social science of psychology.

The academic aspects of student life, and the content and structure of the degree course constituted an important part of the Keele experience, but, there were also other things going on. The late sixties, and especially 1968 was a time of unrest in universities across the world. This partly derived from internal university politics as students were demanding greater representation and freedom within universities. On the wider international scene the Vietnam war and apartheid in South Africa were generating student protest. At Keele there were long, late night debates in the Students' Union and local protest marches. In the middle of June 1968 there was a short sit-in of about 150 students at the university registry building. I went to the debates and a march or two, but not the sit-in.

It feels hard to believe that my undergraduate experience is now forty years in the past. Universities and especially undergraduate degree courses have changed considerably. Studying across the art–science divide is now common place. For a variety of reasons the Foundation Year at Keele no longer exists, one being the now less generous financial support available to present day students. Four year courses lead to greater levels of indebtedness. Also the current expectation that degree courses should provide a stronger support for future employment is in opposition to the kind of liberal education values that were an essential part of the original Keele approach to undergraduate education.

As well as the special characteristics of its degree course, Keele in the mid sixties was also different from other universities in that it was almost wholly residential. It had started off with most of the student accommodation being in the huts which were left over from the previous incarnation of the campus for military training during the second world war. By the time I became a student there was a fair amount of purpose built accommodation. Compared with most students today I think that I had a very privileged experience. I lived on campus for the whole of my four years so there were no problems with difficult landlords. I could walk to lectures rather than having to depend on public transport. The sixties were the days of student grants. I didn't have a full grant but my parents made up the

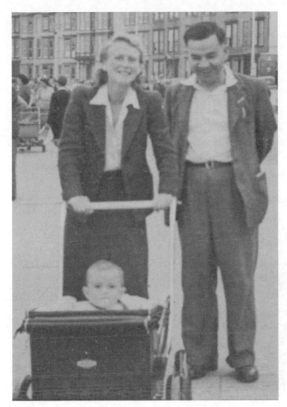

Pram on the prom 1

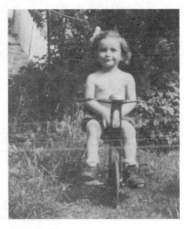

First trike

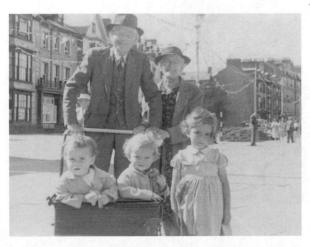

Pram on the prom 2

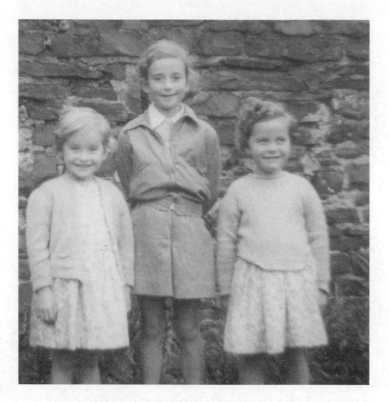

The three of us

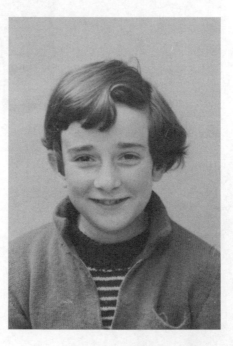

Primary school

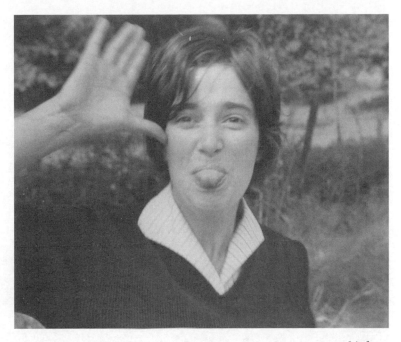

Ya boo

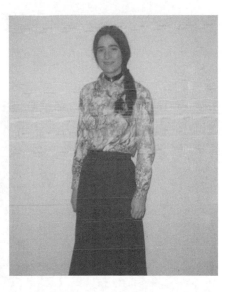

Keele – ready to go out

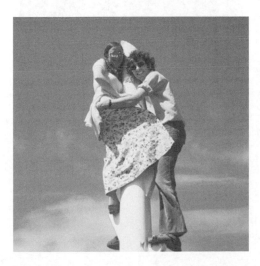

At the lookout

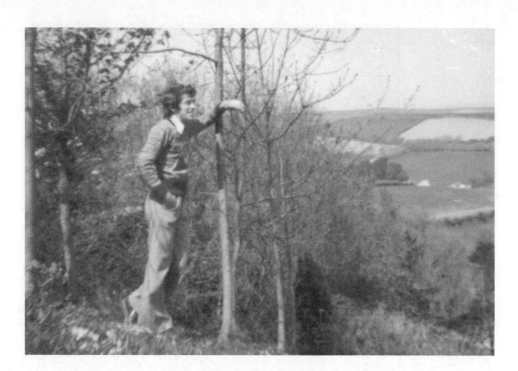

Pete at High Legh

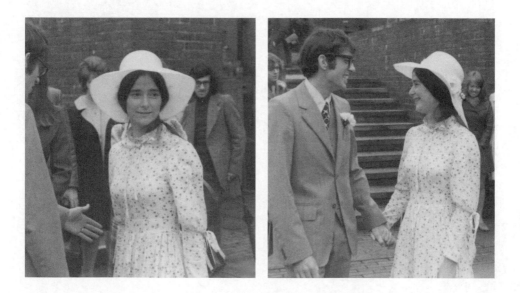

Wedding day
June 24th 1972

difference, and I, along with most of my fellow students, found it easy to live on the amount provided.

Living 'in hall' on campus meant that social contact was also easy. I made friends with other students living in the same hostel building in particular. Closest friends were probably in the same year, but I also got to know others who were a year ahead, which was useful. We met each other particularly at mealtimes, and were provided with almost a surfeit of food – a cooked breakfast was available and then two cooked meals at lunch times and evenings on weekdays. Afterwards we would frequently go for coffee, squeezed into somebody's room. At weekends there was a chance for cooking, in the kitchens provided on each floor, and doing a little 'entertaining'.

As well as cooking, university provided me with my first real experience of having a boyfriend. There were a few shortish relationships, and then one that was more serious and longer-lasting, although with an element of turmoil and, to some extent an 'on/off' quality. Although I kind of knew that this probably wasn't going to make a good long term relationship, I was still upset when we broke up at the beginning of my final year.

In the new calendar year – 1969 – I met Pete and we began 'going around'. In some ways the omens for the two of us were perhaps not that good. An observer might have commented it was a relationship on the 'rebound' – although it never felt like that. Pete told me some time later that he initially asked me out as something of a wager. The issue was whether he, as a second year student, could 'make it' with a final year student – as I was! For both of us though, it was a good relationship from the beginning and we were very much friends, as well as sexual partners. For me our relationship had a degree of ease, comfort and 'rightness' which had been lacking in the previous one.

Of course, one of the perils of beginning a serious relationship towards the end of one partner's undergraduate career is that a degree of separation is almost inevitable. After my graduation in the summer of 1969, I took up a postgraduate place at Lancaster University. It could obviously have been worse, as I had also applied for places at Glasgow and Sussex. Over the next couple of years both of us acquired a degree of familiarity with a particular stretch of the M6. Pete hitch hiked up to Lancaster from Keele. I was lucky to get regular, arranged lifts in the opposite direction.

On this interrupted basis, our relationship became much more serious. As well as making trips up and down the motorway from Keele to Lancaster, we visited my parents in Aberystwyth and got down to Pete's home in rural, coastal North Devon. In many ways his background was different to mine, but in a complicated way. Pete would say it was more working class. His father worked as a shop assistant in the nearby town of Barnstaple. On the other hand he had spent his primary school years at a small local private school.

As the only son of somewhat older parents, the stereotypical expectation could have been that he would be a spoilt and self-centred young person. This was very far from the case. I recognised early on Pete's basic kindness and generosity and this has very definitely continued into maturity. One of his central characteristics is being very generous with his time to other people besides me.

I felt comfortable with Pete's parents and enjoyed his home, a timber built bungalow, set on the hillside above the seaside village of Croyde. The car had to be left at the bottom of the hill, and then you followed the track up through the fields. I found Pete's mother easy to talk to and, in retrospect, I probably owe her a great deal for the way Pete was brought up. Very sadly, she never became my mother-in-law, but I know from one of her letters to Pete that she did approve of me and our relationship. I wish I could have known her better.

Pete and I were together at Keele in the early summer of 1971. We were celebrating the news of his degree results in the refectory. His best friend, Dewi (who, over 35 years later is still one of our closest friends) came to say that the Hall warden wanted a word with him. The news was the worst, Pete's mother had died suddenly of a heart attack at the age of 63. It was a huge shock, but at least his mother had known Pete had achieved his degree. We immediately travelled down to North Devon together to be with Pete's father, and to do the things that had to be done. It was, of course, a difficult time, but I'm sure that being together then helped to reinforce our commitment to each other.

A year after, in the summer of 1972, we were married. Pete was working as an articled clerk in Birmingham and I had a research post at the university. Our first home together was a modern one bedroomed housing association flat in Handsworth Wood which was quite convenient and comfortable.

However, neither of us were enthusiasts for city living, and so when the opportunity arose we were quite keen to move away from Birmingham. In September 1974 I was offered a teaching post at Crewe+Alsager College of Higher Education. This new college was formed after the amalgamation of two previously independent teacher training colleges in the nearby towns of Crewe and Alsager. We moved to the small town, or overgrown village, of Alsager, and bought our first house there. We were becoming reasonably established, and Alsager was to be our home for the next 22 years.

Soon afterwards Pete moved out of accountancy and obtained a research job at Wolverhampton Polytechnic. After eighteen months he moved to a lecturing post at the Further Education college in Crewe. In 1978 the higher level business studies teaching, to which he contributed, was absorbed into Crewe+Alsager College. Consequently we ended up teaching in the same institution, although working on different sites.

Looking back, these were comfortable and enjoyable years. Of course there were periodic frustrations in our jobs, but for me especially this was a largely very satisfying time, developing a new degree course and associated course units, and then getting involved in evaluative research. By then we were well-established in our lives – home, careers, friends and social life.

Then came the realisation that we were coming to the decision not to take the next conventional step. We hadn't actually talked explicitly about it before we were married but when we did start the discussion we found that neither of us had any real desire to have children. We had a very equitable and companionable marriage – we did lots of things together, and we felt that this particular kind of relationship might be more difficult to maintain if there were children on the scene. More fundamentally, and more importantly I have never experienced any real maternal urge. There have been odd occasions when I have speculated on what it might have been like, and how different our lives could have been – but not with any regrets. Since Pete was not keen to experience fatherhood, there was no agonising necessary – not having children just seemed the right decision for *us*.

Though we were absorbed in our lecturing jobs, there was still time for other things. Our social lives revolved largely around the friends we had made at Crewe+Alsager, although through weekend visits we also kept up contact with friends made at university and at school. Beyond that we began to develop (or return to) various activities which helped to keep us occupied on some evenings, weekends, and for parts of our holiday periods.

As already described, I had quite active interests as a child and adolescent. I didn't keep up the roller-skating but we did get out into the countryside to walk when we could. We could easily get out into the countryside immediately around Alsager, although it did not provide the same attractive variety that was available around and about Aberystwyth. However, we were within easy reach of the Peak District, which we soon came to know and enjoy. Getting out there for a day's walking was something that we did quite frequently. Longer expeditions to the Lake District were also easily possible and we had some summer holidays walking in Austria.

I had owned a bike as a teenager but Aberystwyth and its surroundings were too hilly to allow easy cycling, so I had never done much more than a little gentle cycling around the town. Pete, however, had been a keen cyclist and the hills around his home in Devon had not put him off! Pete's argument was that with a good lightweight bike cycling really would be easy – and the Cheshire lanes around and about Alsager did provide good cycling country.

I was persuaded. A good bike did indeed make a huge difference. We cycled quite frequently on fine summer evenings – sometimes with friends, sometimes just the two of us. We would arrange a circuit such that we could have something to eat at a pub, after which there were not too many miles before home. We were lucky in that quite a few such routes, on reasonably quiet roads, were possible, starting out straight from home.

We started to do some easy cycle touring. First we had some weekend rides in areas easily accessible from home. Then we 'graduated' to week long tours during the summer holidays. Our strategy was to take our bikes on the train to the starting town, have a linear tour, and then return by train from our final cycling destination. There was an excitement about travelling from place to place – getting to somewhere new every evening. I enjoyed the relatively leisurely speed at which we cycled (as contrasted with touring by car). It meant that we got a much better appreciation of the countryside, villages and towns through which we travelled. We could also stop very easily whenever there was something interesting to see. We found that we really enjoyed this kind of cycle touring.

Later, we tried cycle touring abroad – in France and Germany. Here we took the very easy option of using companies who provided detailed route information, booked hotels and even transported our luggage from one hotel to the next – the height of cycling luxury! Apart from these useful arrangements, the holidays were very informal – it was certainly not cycling in a regimented group. Usually there tended to be about half a dozen other people doing the same route, at the same time, but you could cycle as independently as you wished. We might meet up with other members of the group now and again during the day, and then had the option to eat together in the evening if we wished. This was a good combination of having some congenial company, but not being 'on top of each other'. It was an interesting and relaxing form of holiday. (Eventually, of course, it was on one such holiday where my MS symptoms first appeared.)

Well, that took care of our summer holidays – but what about the winter? There are many attractions to having something to look forward to during the dark days of winter, and to end a busy term. So we took up skiing! We both like spectacular mountain scenery, and I really enjoy the transformation provided by snow, even in this country. So the combination of these which one finds in ski resorts was a great attraction.

Our first skiing trip was to the Austrian village of Söll. The snow was a little bit on the thin side when we arrived. The nursery slopes just outside the village were not in use and so we had to head up on the chair lift to the higher slopes. This was no loss really as it meant we got a quicker feel for what skiing was all about. The ride up the mountain was magical – above a small chapel perched on a rocky outcrop, a rushing, plunging mountain stream, and then brushing the tops of the pine trees and looking down on the undisturbed snow. The skiing itself was also absorbing and exciting. We felt we were learning quite quickly, and the falling down – of which we did quite a bit – was part of the fun.

Soon after summer was over we enjoyed collecting the next season's ski brochures and beginning the discussion of where to go. We almost wholly confined ourselves to Austrian valley skiing villages, and French purpose built resorts higher up in the mountains. They both had considerable – but quite different – attractions.

One of the pleasures of skiing was that it was all absorbing. One had to – but wanted to anyway – just concentrate on the skiing. You couldn't think about the pile of essays waiting to be marked at home, or the lectures which still had to be prepared for the beginning of the next term. It was an exhilarating, exciting, but also relaxing way of forgetting about worries and deadlines, and so just what was needed at the end of a busy term.

Such was my life before MS. I had been exceedingly fortunate. But did this early period provide any helpful base for the challenges which now faced me? The one thing that was clear was that the easy comfortable life I had taken for granted was going to change. Things would be more uncertain, more difficult. Would I be able to cope?

Chapter Two

Psychologist

Up until July 1993 and the MS diagnosis my life had been a pretty active one. Now I could hardly walk and I was scared to even try getting onto my bike again. The cycling, walking and skiing had been important parts of my life outside of work. I got great enjoyment and satisfaction from them. What would my life be like if these activities were no longer possible?

But I was, and still am, a psychologist. I knew it would be a part of my life that would continue. I also knew that psychology had things to say about identity and threats to identity. I knew that there were social scientists who saw the onset of chronic illness as posing a major disruption, even a 'loss of self'. I also knew that there were other psychologists who had a different, more positive perspective. From early on I hoped that these more positive ideas would help me to cope with the sudden and drastic challenge of becoming chronically ill myself.

Before discussing these coping possibilities I need to go back and make some comment on my experience as a student, and then teacher of psychology. I want to say a little about those aspects of the discipline that I felt were now of quite vital personal relevance.

Psychology at Keele...

Before all this, what had led me into studying psychology in the first place? The major impetus was my decision that I wanted to study at Keele University. As I've indicated, after the first foundation year all the degree courses at Keele were joint honours – you were required to study two subjects. If I had gone to any other university I would have studied Biology. My intention of going to Keele meant that I had to choose a second subject.

A Psychology degree course was then, and still is, quite broad in its intents. The discipline ranges from the biological basis of behaviour at the 'hard' end to (say) counselling approaches at the 'softer' end. The undergraduate degree was (and still is) constrained by the requirements laid down by the British Psychological Society that the whole range of the discipline should be covered.

Thus my memory is of a course in which experimental psychology and the study of the processes of perception, learning and memory were quite central. 'Lab' sessions in which we conducted small scale investigations were also a weekly component of the course. Alongside there were weekly sessions in experimental design and statistical analysis. As well as learning what psychology is all about we needed to gain an understanding of how psychologists go about carrying out research investigations.

As the course progressed, I found that, despite my science background, it was the 'social end' of the discipline that I found the more interesting and intriguing, but also challenging. One of these topics that received minor, almost marginal attention, within my undergraduate degree was the nature of self. Because I think this area of psychology has relevance for my later experiences of coping with disability, I will comment on some of the ideas with which I came into contact at this stage. As will be seen later in the chapter, research and theorising in relation to self has expanded considerably since those days.

Allport, an early contributor in this area, commented that the psychology of personality harbours an 'awesome enigma' – that is 'the problem of self'. So why is it such a problem? Allport stated (and most, if not all readers, would be likely to agree) that each of us has an acute experiential awareness of our own self.

> *The self is something of which we are immediately aware. We think of it as the warm, central, private region of our life. As such it plays a crucial part in our consciousness... Thus it is some kind of core in our being.*[1]

But despite this personal awareness of our own selves it is still difficult to explain exactly what it is we are aware of. Many psychologists, attempting to take a scientific approach within the discipline, were not, at that time, tolerant of such inexactitude. However, there were others who agreed with Allport about the importance of facing up to the enigma.

Another psychologist who attempted to grapple with ideas about, and our experience of, the self was Carl Rogers.[2] He is perhaps better known to non psychologists through his development of client-centred therapy, but it is worth looking at some of the main ideas which contribute to his theory. Rogers came to view self-related processes as being important because his clients in therapy frequently described their experiences and problems in these terms. On the basis of these discussions he developed his *definition of self* as an '...organised, consistent, conceptual gestalt composed of the characteristics of the 'I' or 'me''. Thus his view of self can be described as being global and integrated in character.

In addition Rogers proposes that we each have a view of ourselves as we would like to be – an *ideal self*. Moreover, he suggests that there is a sense in which we are all trying to achieve the best that we can for ourselves. Rogers called this attempt to reach our full potential the *self-actualisation* motive which he saw as being fundamental for all human beings.

Striving towards future realisation of our potential is thus seen to be an important part of our lives. We also have a need for positive feelings about ourselves in the present. Rogers considers that we search for *positive self regard* – that is we need to experience acceptance, warmth, and positive value from significant people in our lives. Such reactions provide comforting feelings of positive success and we feel better about ourselves.

I found these ideas, and those of Allport, interesting. Both psychologists were writing about aspects of personality that seemed to me to be important, and which had personal relevance. At the same time there were clearly limitations and difficulties. These fall into two main categories – those associated with clear definition, and with empirical research.

As already indicated, we are all aware of our own subjective experience of self. It is, though, much more difficult for us to explain just what it is we are aware of. Both authors made some progress in writing about, and clarifying aspects of these experiences. However, there are still limitations and ambiguities in their accounts. For example, what exactly is meant when the self is described as a 'conceptual gestalt' and what is really involved in the self actualisation process?

Both Allport and Rogers were aware of the importance of relevant research. They developed methods which, although not experimental, did allow research into self-related processes and the unique personality. Rogers tape-recorded therapeutic sessions to provide some evidence of the influence of unconditional regard.[3] Allport argued for the value of personal documents in the understanding of personal lives.[4] He reported on one person's life through his examination of the 'Letters of Jenny'. Such methods and research approaches were recognised as valuable by some psychologists but, for the majority in those times, they were seen as going beyond the bounds of what counted as acceptable science.

Some Changes Since...

Psychology as a discipline has, of course, changed quite considerably since the late sixties. As an academic psychologist I have had to follow and keep up with these changes. Indeed, much of the pleasure of an academic career comes from this 'keeping up' and incorporating changes and new developments into one's teaching. In particular, I have been fortunate to be able to follow up my early student interest in self-related processes, and include the topic in my ongoing teaching. It is not possible to chart these changes in any detail within this chapter, or even within the book. This account of changes in psychology is not in any way a comprehensive academic textbook review of the discipline. However, I will make some comment on continuing work in this area for two main reasons.

Firstly, concerns about self and identity have come to have a more direct and immediate personal relevance. Am I (in Christopher Reeve's words) still me?[5] Has my sense of self and identity been interrupted or disrupted? Do I need to re-negotiate a changed sense of who I am? These questions of whether, and to what extent, identity has to be modified are a common theme in both academic and personal accounts of life with chronic illness and disability. My personal responses and reactions will be a part of this continuing commentary on my life.

The second and linked reason for giving issues of self some attention is that these have now become much more important within the discipline. In the 1960s it was rather a fringe interest and not seen as quite respectable by many psychologists. The change in importance and acceptance has derived from changes in the broader discipline. In the 1950s and even into the 1960s psychology was generally defined as the science of *behaviour*. In its attempts to be scientific, psychology focused on behaviour because it could be observed, measured and investigated with some objectivity. But self related processes cannot be observed, definition is problematic and objective investigation was seen as harder still.

What is psychology like now? How has the discipline changed? The briefest description is to say that psychologists now conceive of human beings as 'processors of information' rather than focusing mainly on their observable behaviour. Another summary description which is frequently used is to say that there has been a 'cognitive revolution' in psychology. We are interested in internal cognitions just as much as external behaviour. Behaviour is usually preceded by thoughts of various kinds – problem solving strategies, plans for the future, attitudes, evaluations of ourselves and other people, and so on. If we are to understand and account for behaviour, we also need to understand these internal processes. Psychologists have now developed better ways of investigating such internal cognitions.

But what have been the consequences of these changes in psychology generally and for the study of self related processes in particular? Very briefly, it has enabled the study of the self to move from the sidelines to nearer centre stage. Research and theorising in the area has expanded enormously during the 1980s, 1990s, and into the new millennium. The change from emphasising behaviour to emphasising cognitions allows us to see the self in terms of (just) another set of cognitions, rather than a vague, elusive construction which is difficult to define precisely and investigate.

This much expanded interest has led to some of the issues touched on above, in relation to Rogers' thinking, being re-addressed.

One Self or Many?

As indicated, Carl Rogers viewed the self as being global and unitary in character – an integrated 'gestalt'. Hazel Markus has been one of the most important proponents of the more recent cognitive approach to self related processes.[6] The nub of his position is that just as we have conceptions, or schemas, of the objects or events in the external world, so we also have schemas about ourselves and our own personal behaviour. This view of self is essentially multiple and differentiated. We have many different schemas about ourselves which represent different aspects or facets of the person which each of us is.

Thus, the self is seen as a set of self-schemas. Each schema is gradually built up by the individual to summarise, explain and understand their own ongoing experience in a particular context. Such schemas might be quite general (e.g. 'I am a generous person' or 'I am creative'), but are quite likely to be more specific and idiosyncratic (e.g. 'I am quite talkative in the company of two or three others, but shy in larger groupings').

As with any schema, self-schemas not only summarise information but are also involved in the processing of new information, and the management of ongoing behaviour. So the last person mentioned above might tend to seek out smaller, more intimate groupings on social occasions. Also, different schemas will be at the forefront of our minds at different times, and in different places. Markus refers to working schemas, or the working self-concept.

Another parallel way of thinking about multiple conceptions of who we are is through the allied concept of identity. It is a concept which is used by psychologists and sociologists, but it is also one that is centre stage in modern life and discourse. Very few of us are now likely to avoid any engagement with the identity question 'Who am I?'. Self-schemas are likely, to a degree, to be implicit; identity statements are more likely to be explicit. Indeed one strategy which social scientists have used to investigate identity is to ask people to give, say 20 answers to the question 'Who am I?' Most people do not have any great difficulty in dealing with this kind of task because we have already provided our own answers for ourselves and use them in such social situations as introducing ourselves to new people at parties.

Baumeister effectively sees answers to the question 'who am I?' as providing the units of self-definition or identity components.[7] Thus, statements such as 'I am a psychologist, a teacher, a cyclist, and I am Welsh and a woman' are identity statements which contribute to defining who I am.

Baumeister suggests that these identity components fulfil important functions for us. One of these is that they support our sense of differentiation from others. In other words they bolster our sense of individuality and uniqueness – they tell us who we are. Secondly, our sense of identity provides us with feelings of continuity over time – the feeling of being the same person today as yesterday, or last year. Thus, Baumeister argues that a clearly worked out sense of identity has advantages.

These ideas emphasise a multiple view of self. They may not be suggesting that we have many separate selves, but certainly that there are separate facets of self. It is being proposed that we have a differentiated view of ourselves and that this has many advantages.

A Degree of Integration?

So, is there still a concern for a more integrated, unitary representation of self? At a subjective level I would think that many of us would want to claim that we experience a degree of integration. But how can this integration be represented and explained more formally? There are a number of possible sources of such integration.

In 'everyday' non specialist discussion about self, the idea of self-esteem is likely to make a contribution. This has also been an important idea for psychologists. It seems to have a global character to it. Popular writing often suggests that people have generally high esteem (or not). But this kind of global self-evaluation is not a straightforward matter.

The earlier discussion, and our own experience, would suggest that we evaluate different aspects of ourselves. We might think that we are doing pretty well in relation to one area of performance, but less well in others. Can we put these various assessments together to arrive at some overall self evaluation? There is dispute among psychologists as to whether this happens, and if there is some 'putting together' about how this could be organised. So, the idea of general self-esteem is probably not quite as straightforward as it is sometimes assumed to be.

Another meaning of the term self-esteem involves a concern with general self-acceptance. The primary reaction here is emotional, rather than cognitive. It is to do with liking rather than evaluating ourselves, and it is inherently global and holistic. It is probably most usually accepted that we like someone else as a whole, rather than in part. We make an overall, emotional judgement about their worth.

It has been argued by quite a number of psychologists over the years that we make similar judgements about ourselves. We make global assessments of our own self-worth. Positive self-acceptance means that we generally tend to like and accept ourselves in spite of various faults and limitations. We are likely to agree with statements such as 'I feel that I am a person of worth – as good as anybody else' or 'In spite of my faults I am generally satisfied with the kind of person I am'. It is argued that positive self-acceptance derives from warm, supportive and accepting relationships with important caretakers, in early life in particular.

One of the psychologists who attempts to reconcile such a model of global self-acceptance with the multiple accounts of self discussed earlier is Seymour Epstein.[8] He sees overall self-acceptance (or lack of it) as providing the apex of a hierarchy of more specific views of different aspects of self. These more specific views can be seen as similar to the schemas or identity statements referred to earlier. Epstein's account adds to those of Markus and Baumeister in that he proposes that such self-statements are organised into a hierarchical and reasonably integrated, but implicit self-system.

Further, he argues that such a system can be seen as comprising a self *theory*. The proposal is that just as scientists develop theories about the world around them / us, each of us develops a theory about who we are and our place in the world. Epstein argues that each of us requires such a theory to make sense of our ongoing self related experience and to manage our personal behaviour, although the theory is partly implicit and unlikely to be fully conscious.

A rather different and more recent perspective on integration involves the proposal that one useful way of portraying aspects of self is in terms of personal narrative.[9] The proposal here is that we have an ongoing need to tell our own story – to other people, but also to ourselves. That story will, at least partly, be about our own personal experiences, about the things – big and small – which happen to us. It will also be about how we react to and cope with these happenings and events and use our own personal resources to do so.

Within such a story or narrative there is a requirement for continuity – it needs to be the *same* story, but there is also a need for change and revision as new events and experiences occur. These may well add to or extend the story as time passes. However, there is also likely to be a need to incorporate inconsistencies in experience or even events which have the potential to disrupt the story. We want to construct a coherent, integrated story of ourselves and our experience.

Aspects of Self-Management

The idea of goal setting is an important one. It emphasises that the self system has motivational connections. One of the most comprehensive and well-developed contributions in this area comes in Bandura's model of self-regulatory processes.[10] He argues that through childhood and into adulthood we learn to set standards for our own behaviour and achievement – self standards in all sorts of areas of our lives.

We learn these through admonition and example by powerful others – parents, teachers, heroes or models of various kinds. Bandura proposes that without such standards and consequent evaluative involvement in their achievement we run the risk of being bored and unmotivated and dependent on external sources of excitement. On the other hand if we tend to set standards which are too high – that is standards which we are not often able to actually achieve – then we can become discouraged and depressed.

Effective self-management is best achieved when we are able to set appropriate goals and standards for ourselves, standards which are demanding – but not too demanding. It also helps if we can organise goals which are specific, short term and achievable. Then we can celebrate and reward ourselves for our success. Bandura calls this kind of self-reward self-reinforcement and it is an important motivator within his proposed system. Ideally, specific standards and short term goals contribute towards longer term, more ambitious targets, but provide us with feelings of success and achievement along the way.

In this abbreviated description there is a danger that such a system can appear too rational to represent our more messy and emotional experiences of actual achievement or the lack of it. But rewards and failures surely do link to the real pleasures and pains of our ongoing personal plans and ambitions within our lives.

Markus has extended his ideas about self-schemas in a way which perhaps gives a better indication of what motivational experiences actually feel like. He suggests that it is useful to think of what he calls possible selves.[11] They represent the 'future oriented components of the self-system'. They can summarise what we want to become, but also what we are afraid of becoming, mental 'pictures' of, say, a successful, loved, or physically fit self, but perhaps also a clumsy, or helpless self. Vivid, imagined representations of such different possibilities can provide powerful, quite detailed, and emotionally salient goal possibilities which we will then work towards, or try to avoid if they represent negative selves

Selves in the Social Context

So far this account has had a somewhat individualistic emphasis. There has not been much reference to the roles and influences of other people. There has perhaps been a past tendency for some psychologists to neglect the social context. The study of self tended to be positioned as part of the study of personality which in turn has been placed under the heading of the study of *individual* differences.

But now the study of personality has become much more social and cognitive in character.[12] This is certainly true of our current thinking about self-processes. How could it be otherwise? Much of our ongoing self-related experience takes place in relation to, and in the context of others. There may not actually be another person present, but still our thinking is likely to involve a hypothetical other person. Self is essentially and necessarily social in character. This social dimension to the self has come to be seen as crucial. But it is also complex and ambiguous, influenced by social conventions and by the wider cultural context.

One of the most obvious aspects of this social influence that we all experience is the social feedback we receive from others. In our early years most of us who are fortunate will have been at the centre of much direct, primarily positive reaction from parents and other significant others. As we get older more of the feedback is quite likely to be less direct and often ambiguous in character – it will need to be interpreted. But this feedback is still important to our ongoing feelings about ourselves.

Another social evaluation process in which we engage is that of social comparison.[13] We want to know how we are doing in comparison with others in relation to various aspects of our lives and achievements. Can we evaluate ourselves as being superior to our 'comparison others', or are we doing less well? A crucial question both for us individually, and as an issue for psychologists, is that of who we choose to compare ourselves with. Psychological investigation suggests that it will most usually be others who are reasonably like ourselves as this will yield the most useful information. Though in our consumer oriented world there is much pressure on us to make aspirational comparisons, and that is not always beneficial to our well-being.

Two other aspects of selves in the social context have a more direct implication for social interaction. These are self-presentation and self-disclosure. There is a degree of tension between these two sets of processes.

There are many social situations, perhaps especially when we are meeting people for the first time, when most of us would want to give a good impression of ourselves. We are likely to use various tactics of impression management to do this. We put on the best positive act that we can, with appropriate supporting props, while concealing more negative characteristics. Goffman was a sociologist who used this kind of analogy with acting and the theatre to support his account of self-presentational processes.[14] Although it is important not to overact in case one gets found out there is an emphasis on presenting the best image. There is evidence that people do indeed change their behaviour to create an impression when they know that others are observing them.

Positive self-presentation is likely to be advantageous when we need to make an impression. However, appropriate self-disclosure is more important as relationships begin and develop.[15] As the term suggests, disclosure can involve revealing less desirable as well as more positive characteristics or experiences. Thus, there are risks involved. But, appropriately paced and reciprocal disclosure of increasingly intimate information plays an essential role in the forming of close relationships. Such disclosure can make one vulnerable but if there is positive reaction it can support and validate feelings and knowledge about oneself and therefore be rewarding in a fundamental way.

Our sense of self-identity is also socially rooted in the groups to which we belong.[16] These may be relatively small groups of which we have a personal and actual membership, such as the local hockey team, or stamp collecting society. In addition there will be broader social groupings or categories; we will each belong to various ones, such as being a European, a socialist, a reader of the *Guardian*. Obviously, different groupings will be salient for different individuals.

To a degree, part of our sense of identity and self-esteem derives from the groups to which we belong. This can perhaps be seen most readily in the reactions of the football supporter whose team has won. Even though he is a supporter, not a player, the team's success is *his* success also. At a somewhat more abstract level many of us could perhaps imagine circumstances in which we would take pride in being a European against, say, an American.

But there are some social psychologists who give social influences on self greater prominence than has been suggested so far. Indeed they argue that continually changing social experience, in a whole variety of social situations, means that any kind of stable self has only limited existence. Our sense of self, it is proposed, is likely to change quite considerably over time and varying contexts and in different relationships. In this view, social influence can be so great that it has a dominating, but changing influence on self-perception so that self is primarily fluid in character and that

> We come to be aware that each truth about ourselves is a construction of the moment, true only for a given time and within certain relationships.[17]

In this interpretation, it is almost the case that self hardly has any real, stable existence. Of course, change does occur in response to changing circumstances, but others (including myself) would argue that self related cognitions do have some continuing existence with at least a degree of stability.

It should be evident though that there cannot be some 'thing' that corresponds to the self. To refer at all to *the* self is deceptive. Instead, each of us is operating with a set of self-related schemas that contribute to a complex self-system. These complex self-processes constitute part of each person's cognitive system for making sense of themselves and the world around them. Thus, we view our personal world through, and in terms of, the implicit theory we have negotiated about ourselves.

There are tensions and oppositions within the system and the way that it operates. There is tension between the multiple, varied and differentiated schemas we have about aspects of ourselves, but also the pressure towards some degree of integration and unity. The system is also a dynamic and changing one in response to new, ongoing experience and social interaction. At the same time there are advantages to maintaining a degree of continuing stability.

Psychological Research Methods: Some Changing Emphases...

Earlier in this chapter I referred to 'doing' psychology – Psychology is necessarily about carrying out investigations, and it is through these that the knowledge content of the discipline is accumulated. Thus, the empirical inquiry methods used to carry out that research are of central concern within the discipline. Psychology has been seen as a scientific discipline and thus one that uses scientific research methods. A scientific approach provides the basis for the production of agreed, objective research findings leading to the development of well-based theoretical understanding. Taking a scientific approach within psychology has the advantage of allowing the discipline to emulate the prestigious and successful physical sciences.

Of course, from the early days, and as the discipline developed, there were always some whose work did not coincide with this dominant perspective. Freud's work could clearly not be seen as fitting within the confines of a conventional scientific approach. Later, Rogers and others argued that a narrow scientific approach could not cope adequately with the real complexities of human behaviour, emotions and adjustment. Greater flexibility and less rigidity of method was required.

As an undergraduate, despite my scientific background, I did have some sympathy with the methodological concerns briefly identified above. Not that I thought that an experimental, scientific approach was altogether inappropriate, but rather that something more, or in addition, was needed. However, the problem then was that alternative methods did not seem to have been worked out with sufficient clarity and detail.

Matters have changed since. Much of my teaching career has been spent working quite closely with sociologists. I soon found out that many sociologists have had longer term, more substantial and well worked out criticism of a scientific approach as a way of making sense of human behaviour and society. Briefly, they have argued that experiments can over-simplify and distort the human responses that they are trying to investigate. Researchers can spend too much time trying to measure the unmeasurable. Instead, sociologists have argued in favour of the importance of trying to *understand* human responses and action. They have argued for the value of qualitative, interpretive and more open-ended research approaches such as unstructured interviews and participant observation. The objective is to find the meanings behind the actions.

Many sociologists (and now quite a few psychologists) would see qualitative, interpretive approaches as being superior to the scientific, quantitative, and especially experimental approach. More would now accept that methods derived from both approaches have their value, partly depending on the problem being investigated, but also because they provide different kinds of insights into the human condition.[18]

It is certainly true that the use of qualitative methods has expanded considerably across the social sciences in recent years. You can no longer count yourself as a properly educated researcher unless you have some knowledge, and probably experience as well, of qualitative methods. Within psychology both post-graduate, and undergraduate level textbooks on the use of qualitative methods have been published.[19]

Part of the reason for the expansion and change in emphasis is that for many researchers the argument that qualitative methods can make an important research contribution has been won. A second reason is that procedures for analysing qualitative data have improved. Computer software for analysing qualitative, as well as quantitative data is now tested and available.

Controversy about methods and methodology within psychology has not disappeared. Quite properly, there is continuing discussion – and argument. But now, there is clearly a greater range of available methods which have achieved wider, if not full acceptance within the discipline.

Health Psychology…

The cognitive influence and the increased acceptance of a plurality of research approaches are certainly not the only changes in the discipline of psychology that have happened since the 1960s. Another kind of change has been the emergence of new areas of interest and research within the discipline.

One such area which didn't really exist at all back in the 1960s, but which has now come to have quite a strong presence within the discipline, is health psychology. The basic rationale for the development of this area has been that health and illness have a psychological as well as a bodily dimension. Persuading people to safeguard their health (e.g. eating healthily, taking exercise, stopping smoking) is, in many ways, a psychological matter. Coping with illness, even at the mundane level (for instance deciding whether to take the medicine) also involves psychological aspects.

Health psychology has expanded enormously over the past ten to fifteen years in a number of ways. Firstly, an expanded number of topics and areas which are of relevance to health psychology have been identified and are being researched. Secondly, and associated with this, a substantial number of academic journals publishing health psychology research have been founded. Thirdly, there is now a qualification route through which one can become a health psychologist. Lastly, the number of post-graduate courses in health psychology linked to this qualification procedure has increased substantially. Employment opportunities are also expanding.

My own contact with health psychology has come at two points. At the end of the 1980s the college department in which I taught established a set of multidisciplinary course units in health studies (including sociology of health as well as health psychology, and also educational and philosophical aspects). I was asked to contribute to the teaching of health psychology and therefore I had to 'read up' on the area to do this.

For various reasons this contribution lasted only for two or three years and then other people took over the teaching. However, when I developed MS my interest in the area was reawakened – at a more personal level. Investigation of the literature on chronic illness provided some interesting material. A pervasive and, I think, appropriate theme was that of chronic illness as a disrupter of identity. However, my reaction as someone who had a chronic illness was that the discussions could be rather too negative and pessimistic.

Another important outcome of this further investigation of the health psychology literature related to methodological issues. It became clear that although there was much research in this area which proceeded along traditional lines (i.e. taking a largely scientific approach) there was also a strong interest in qualitative, interpretive possibilities. This is hardly surprising. As one part of the quest to know more about the psychology of illness, we surely need to understand the *experience* of illness. The best way to do this is to use qualitative research methods to ask people what it *feels* like.

As part of this qualitative emphasis there has been an interest in the 'storied nature of health and illness'.[20] The experience of chronic illness in particular takes place over time – adjustment to it, and management of it is an ongoing process. Thus the stories people tell of their own ongoing illness experience can provide important sources of understanding. Those stories are also obviously important to the people who tell them. Constructing the story is an important part of the adjustment and management process. It provides an opportunity to overcome the disruption to identity which has been posed by the illness experience and to develop a renewed, readjusted self-narrative.

This book provides an account of my own readjusted self-narrative as well as a commentary on the challenge of more practical aspects of coping with chronic illness and disability.

Notes and References

1. Alport, G. (1961). *Pattern and Growth in Personality*. New York: Holt, Rinehart and Winston.
2. Rogers, C.R. (1951). *Client-centered Therapy; Its current practice, implications and theory*. Boston: Houghton.
3. For example in Rogers, C.R. & Dymond, R.F. (Eds.) *Psychotherapy and Personality Change: Co-ordinated studies in the client-centered approach*. Chicago: University of Chicago Press.
4. Allport, G. (1965). *Letters from Jenny*. New York: Harcourt, Brace, Jovanovich.
5. From Christopher Reeve's autobiography. Reeve, C. (1998). *Still Me*. London: Century.
6. Markus has made a major contribution to research and theorising in this area. An early article which introduced the concept of a self-schema was Markus, H. (1977). Self-schemata and processing information about the self. *Journal of Personality and Social Psychology*, 35, 63-78.

7. Baumeister provides an accessible account of his ideas about the nature of identity in Baumeister, R.F., (1986). *Identity: Cultural Change and the Struggle for Self*. New York: Oxford University Press.

8. Epstein, S. (1973). The self-concept revisited, *or* a theory of a theory. *American Psychologist*, 28, 404-416.

9. One of the major contributors to narrative psychology is McAdams: McAdams, D. P. (1997). *Stories We Live By: Personal myths and the making of the self*. New York: Guilford Press.

10. The major text here is Bandura, A. (1986). *Social Foundations of Thought and Action*. Englewood Cliffs, New Jersey: Prentice-Hall.

11. Markus, H. & Nurius, P. (1986). Possible selves. *American Psychologist*, 41, 954-969.

12. Of course, the social conception of self goes back a long way – especially through sociological contributions. Cooley's idea of the 'looking glass self' was an early influential model. Cooley, C.H. (1902). *Human Nature and the Social Order*. New York: Scribners.

13. Early contributions derive from the work of Leon Festinger. Festinger, L. (1954). A theory of social comparison processes. *Human Relations*, 7, 117-140. More recent, more sophisticated thinking comes in the extensive work of Tesser and Campbell, for example, Tesser, A.& Campbell, J.(1982). Self evaluation maintenance and the perception of friends and strangers. *Journal of Personality*. 50, 261-279.

14. Goffman, E. (1959) *The Presentation of Self in Everyday Life*. New York: Doubleday & Co.

15. A reasonably accessible review is provided in Derlega, V.J., Metts, S., Petronio, S. and Margulis, S,T. (1993). *Self-Disclosure*. London: Sage.

16. A good text-book summary of relevant ideas is provided in Brown, H. (1985). *People, Groups and Society*. Milton Keynes: Open University Press.

17. This quotation is taken from Gergen, K. (1991). *The Saturated Self: Dilemmas of Identity in Contemporary Life*. New York: Basic Books, p. 16.

18. See, for example, Bryman, A (1988). *Quantity and Quality in Social Research*. London: Unwin Hyman Ltd.

19. For example, Smith, J.A., Harre, R. & Van Langenhove, L. (1995). *Rethinking Methods in Psychology*. London: Sage.

20. Murray, M. (1999). The storied nature of health and illness. In M. Murray & K. Chaimberlain (Eds), *Qualitative Health Psychology*. London: Sage.

Chapter Three

An Innovative Career?

In 1974 I was looking for a new lecturing post. One of my applications was for a post at Crewe+Alsager College of Higher Education. This college was then a teacher training institution. It had just been formed by the amalgamation of two previously separate colleges at Crewe (of railway fame) and Alsager, towns about five miles apart. I had some applications in for university posts, but it was the Crewe+Alsager post that attracted me most. I accepted their job offer with enthusiasm.

What was it that made me want this particular post? Although the information provided was rather sketchy, it was clear that some new developments were in the offing. Colleges that had previously provided just teacher training were now to offer a new two year qualification, a Diploma in Higher Education (or Dip. H.E.). This would be the equivalent of the first two years of a degree, but would be broader and less specialised in nature.

I was appointed to contribute to this development at the newly constituted Crewe+Alsager College of Higher Education. I would teach within the social sciences, but there were plans to support the development of student skills. I would have the opportunity to take part in some new teaching initiatives. It sounded both interesting and exciting.

When I arrived at Alsager (where most of my teaching took place) I found I was a member of a small group of new tutors. I would work alongside a second young psychologist. There were also two newly appointed sociologists and two philosophers. I was pleased that I would become a member of such a multidisciplinary group. I had never been the kind of psychologist (and there are, or certainly were some) who saw psychology as superior to the other social science disciplines.

Right from the start I found Crewe+Alsager a friendly place to work. In those more relaxed days in higher education everybody was usually free from teaching at mid morning. Most tutors would take coffee in the senior common room. Consequently there was a chance to chat to many of the established tutors, as well as members of 'our' newly appointed group.

Inevitably, there were also some tensions and perhaps prejudices. We were 'Brian's Lions'. Brian Milner was the relatively young philosopher who was already in post when we arrived. He was in charge of the disciplines underlying education, and had had a great deal to do with establishing our appointments. We were the first tutors who had not gone through the usual 'apprenticeship' of having substantial school teaching experience prior to appointment. As well as having undergone the merger of two previously independent colleges, the new institution was facing the challenge of extending its courses beyond those which were solely involved with teacher training.

To begin with we had to earn our way by teaching on existing courses. At that time intending teachers were expected to study the psychology, sociology and philosophy of education. Our new group contributed to this teaching. But our main objective was to plan a submission to the Council for National Academic Awards (the CNAA). This was the body which then approved higher education courses in those institutions that were not part of the university sector. The submission would constitute a DipHE in Human Behavioural Studies involving course units in psychology, sociology, philosophy and others which concentrated on skill development.

It has long been argued that degree students acquire various high level cognitive skills as a by-product of their academic studies. These are skills such as those of problem identification, library skills, analysis, argument, etc. Such skills are likely to be of considerable value to students as they enter employment.

The underlying rationale of the proposed package was that it would place a more direct emphasis upon important cognitive and interpersonal skills. In other words skills that had previously been seen as an almost automatic by-product of the academic process would now have more direct attention. The emphasis on skills in the undergraduate curriculum has now become much more commonplace, but back in the mid 1970s it was definitely pioneering.

The most conventional of the course units which contributed to the 'skills package' was a social science research methods unit. This kind of unit has always contributed to psychology and sociology degree courses. It is skill oriented in the sense that students have to acquire the skills of doing research.

Two other course units were more unusual. The names of the units give some indication of their aims and the skill areas involved. They were Reason and Argument and Communication and Group Behaviour. The first of these focused on strategies for constructing effective arguments, and also with the evaluation of other people's arguments. Its content was largely drawn from philosophy, but with a focus on application.

The second unit concentrated on interpersonal and group related skills. Both ordinary social life but also our working lives require us to work effectively with other people. This unit had the purpose of helping students to get a better general understanding of the interpersonal skills involved, but also a more particular appreciation of their own strengths and weaknesses in this area. This unit drew primarily on a psychological base.

The fourth unit was a project unit. Students completed a small piece of applied research for themselves, so using the skills previously acquired.

This set of course units, which made up the overall programme in Human Behavioural Studies, gained CNAA approval in April 1978. We admitted our first students the following September. The programme was a flexible one that allowed a fair degree of student choice of course units. The basic requirement was that students should complete sets of course units, in two subject areas out of psychology, sociology, philosophy and the skills units (which had the uninspiring name of Development Studies).

We were pleased and excited to have the programme fully approved. It was good to have our own students, rather than just providing service teaching for students involved in teacher training. However, we soon discovered that the process of submitting course programmes for approval was not over. The national plan for the DipHE was that it would provide a qualification in its own right, but it became clear that many of our students would prefer to obtain a degree. This level of qualification continued to have the greater reputation. As tutors we also accepted this conventional position. We wanted to take things further and offer a degree rather than just a DipHE. The next question was, what kind of degree was desirable and possible?

Going Independent…

The most obvious and straightforward possibility was that of providing third year course units in psychology, sociology and philosophy to provide a full degree in human behavioural studies. However, we soon found that there were difficulties. At the end of the seventies, we required permission from a regional committee in order to put on any new degree courses. This was a time before the major expansion in student numbers of more recent years. The authorities wanted to avoid 'over provision' in particular subject areas. We soon found that we could not obtain approval for putting forward a new final year programme which involved course units in psychology, sociology or philosophy.

So, what other route could we find to achieve a third year 'top-up' to the Dip.H.E.? The strategy we adopted was an ambitious one. It was to develop and enlarge the project unit out of the already approved skills package. This would become the major part of the final year of our proposed degree and constitute a B.A. by Independent Study.

Our rationale for this proposal derived from the huge recent increases in the knowledge content of degree disciplines. It is impossible for an undergraduate to cover all of this content. It is more important that students acquire the skills needed to address and work through problems and topics which they have not previously faced. Skills such as problem identification and analysis, literature search and evaluation then become crucial and central.

Consequently, in their final year, instead of concentrating on acquiring more knowledge, students would research into a topic of their own choosing. They would investigate their topic through library work, but most likely they would also carry out some empirical work, or have a placement with a social organisation. An important part of the rationale for independent study is that students are likely to best develop these high level skills and capabilities by being expected to take real responsibility for working independently on a challenging project. Within such a programme skill acquisition is necessarily integral to the teaching of the degree rather than being any kind of separate 'add-on'.

Our proposal was quite an ambitious and innovative one. It was not completely new. Two other degrees with similar approaches had just gained approval, although with a degree of difficulty in both cases. These were at the then Polytechnic of North East London, and at Lancaster University. But ours would be just the third degree of this kind out of all the undergraduate degrees across the country – so making it quite a rarity. We didn't intend that our degree by independent study would follow exactly the same pattern of the other two. It would have its own special character.

The next challenge was to achieve approval from the CNAA – quite a daunting process. We had to provide a clear rationale for the programme with comment on teaching strategies and procedures for maintaining degree standards. We prepared an extensive document containing all this information and sent it off to the CNAA. The final part of the procedure was to face a panel of eminent academics for what was effectively an oral examination of our proposal.

To our great disappointment we were not successful at this first validation event, but we received some positive encouragement. So, we set to making suitable adjustments. The second time round, a year later, we were successful. and had a party of tutors and students to celebrate. As tutors we felt very pleased with ourselves indeed. We had achieved the validation of an innovatory and unconventional degree at a college which until that point had had limited experience of any kind of degree level work.

We had also gained experience of working closely together on an important long-term, challenging project, cementing a strong sense of group identity. We knew each other pretty well – warts and all. There were, of course, stresses and strains, but all of us felt a very positive pride in what we had achieved, and a real sense of group cohesion and loyalty.

What Kind of Degree?

The essential feature of the degree – that students would complete a major independent project in their final year – has been described.

However, the organisation of the degree and the teaching arrangements required for its success are obviously complex. Students cannot 'do' a project just like that. They need help and support during the earlier years of the degree to lead up to this final year challenge.

We were lucky in our first cohort of very enthusiastic students who did manage their degrees with less support than was probably desirable – they were well into their DipHE course before the complete degree programme was validated. Important procedures for supporting students in the development of their project ideas did already exist within the validated degree. But it was also the case that many improvements resulted from our experience as we actually implemented the programme. Thus the brief description of the operation of the programme which follows outlines the arrangements which existed after the degree had been running for a number of years.

By this time the degree had undergone some expansion in terms of the subject areas that contributed to the programme. Students could now select units in health studies, special education and youth and community studies as well as the original psychology, sociology and philosophy. These additional possibilities clearly identified the degree programme as being rooted in the applied social sciences. Real world practical problems were an important focus within the degree. We gave our degree a more informative title. It was now a BA in Applied Social Studies by Independent Study.

But how exactly could we help our students so that they would be able to confront the challenges of their third year? There were two main 'strands' to our preparatory process. Firstly, as already outlined, we placed considerable emphasis on the acquisition of the necessary research skills. Secondly, students worked on developing a detailed project proposal before they reached their third year.

From early on, and certainly from the end of the first year, we encouraged students to think forward to their third year project. We expected them to begin to develop an 'ideas file'. This would include, for example, jottings, newspaper cuttings, references, contact names. It would provide a source of possibilities and inspiration for the further development of project ideas. During the second year, in consultation with tutors, students were required to work more formally on this development process.

The culmination of this, at the end of the spring term, was the submission, by each student, of an initial project proposal document. This set out in some considerable detail the aims and expected components of the project. Any practical research work or placements had to be sorted out as far as possible at this stage. Students also needed to demonstrate their awareness of the relevant academic literature.

We required such a thorough document because it would form a contract for a major part of the student's final year programme. Although the exact maximum size of a student's independent project has varied a little over the years, an indication of its significance derives from the fact that it could constitute up to five sixths, or close to 80% of final year assessed work, and be up to 30,000 words in length.

Students used the detailed tutor feedback on the provisional proposal to develop a final proposal. They then submitted this to a formal 'Registration Board' that met in the latter part of the summer term. The registration board included all tutors on the degree, but also tutors from other departments in the college, and outside academics and practitioners. It was an important part of the process of confirming the standard of the degree – to the validating body, the outside world including employers, and to the students themselves. When they had their proposal accepted by the Registration Board, and all second year course units completed, students were ready to enter the third year of their degree programme.

Students and Projects…

So what kind of projects did students complete? In order to work successfully on a project through their final year students needed to identify a problem area in which they had a strong interest. Such interests could develop for a number of reasons. Some students would link their project area to their intended career. Others might want to contribute to work on a particular social problem, or take ideas from their own personal experience, and for some a more traditional academic concern where they found something interesting for its own sake.

What were the essential characteristics of an independent project? It was likely to involve a problem oriented investigation into a given topic area, consist of a number of inter-related component essays, and would probably also include practical work of some kind. Case studies, interviews, observation and placements were more common than experimental investigations. An independent project should be more than a straightforward text book summary. Originality and individuality were likely to derive from problem orientation and especially the investigation of a particular example, or local situation.

Even without going into any detail of content a few project titles might give some hint of the kind of issues that our students tackled:

- Trans-racial Adoption: Problems, Perspectives and the Policy Debate.
- The Psychology of Adapting to Blindness.
- Prisons: Punishment or Rehabilitation.
- Careers Guidance for People with Special Needs.

Many of our students chose projects which, to a greater or lesser degree, had a personal relevance in their lives, this being advantageous in many ways. We judged that such intrinsic interest had a valuable role in supporting overall student motivation. As one student put it "You have to be 'into' your project, because if you're not you won't have the dedication or the commitment to push yourself into finding out the answers to the questions you are asking." On the other hand students had to be counselled to avoid pre-judgement and bias. It is an indicator of good students that they are able to retain appropriate objectivity in spite of their personal interest.

Evaluation…

Maybe the degree was interesting and innovative, but was it successful, did it work in practice, did students appreciate it? Evaluating any educational practice is a complicated business. The best approach is to gather information from a number of sources.

The most obvious approach to evaluating a degree is finding out what the customers, the students, think. From the beginning we held informal end of term discussions with our students, doing our best to encourage them to give their honest reactions – negative as well as positive. We also used more formal questionnaires. A 1994 survey of student opinion, had a response rate of over 80%, with generally positive reactions. For example, the great majority agreed with the statement that 'I have enjoyed the challenge of exploring a project area which I have chosen for myself'. Most wrote that they were pleased to be completing a degree by independent study. Even if the 20% of students who didn't complete the survey might have tended towards more negative perceptions, this provides a largely enthusiastic picture.

Open ended comment from students reinforces this perception. The strongest impression given by the students is of a great sense of achievement at the completion of the third year independent project:

> *I found this final independent study year very hard work but also very rewarding with a real sense of achievement on the completion of my project.*

I definitely look back on the year with a sense of achievement, primarily drawn from the feeling that I overcame difficulties well...Knowing that the independent study was my responsibility and mine alone gave me the incentive to make it good.

I feel a great sense of achievement and, despite the hard work, a sense of regret that it has ended. Overall, this was a tremendous experience that I wouldn't have missed for the world.[1]

The majority of such free comment was positive, although the above probably represent the more eloquent. But there were also comments that represented greater difficulty, or real struggle in coping with the demands of the final year.

The second source of evaluation was from external experts. Most importantly we had the regular reactions of our external examiners who came from suitable departments in other universities. It was their job to be critical whenever that was necessary, but they usually had positive comment also. One external examiner, for example, wrote that

...The dissertations are...difficult to compare with those of other institutions...Whilst some were rather poor overall, others were excellent in their coverage of the literature and often presented interesting theoretical analyses which compared favourably with some master's theses.

These days, of course, more formal quality audits of university courses take place. In 1991, for example we were visited by Her Majesty's Inspectors (HMIs). The report commented that students were gradually introduced to an independent study approach in a way that ensured 'a rigorous and educationally valid approach to self managed learning'. The inspectors commented that the projects of many who received a 1st class or 2.1 degree were worthy of publication, or the award of a higher degree.

A Degree of Reflection...

So, from the foregoing, it should be evident that the experience of being involved in the instigation and development of an independent study degree has been personally important and has given me considerable satisfaction and a sense of achievement in my career. However, this book is primarily about reactions to, and the management of my coping with, MS. Has the experience of working on an independent study degree had any kind of impact on this more recent part of my life?

Though it perhaps seems rather unlikely, there has actually been some considerable benefit, particularly through the experience of developing and teaching on one of the units which contributed to our degree by independent study. The relevant unit was 'Communication and Group Behaviour' which, as mentioned previously, focussed on personal and social skills. This unit, along with some others in the degree, drew upon the process of reflection, and it is this concern with, and attention to, reflection and reflective skills, which has been of particular importance.

First of all, some brief comment on this term 'reflection' and the attention it has received recently in the context of higher education and social practice is appropriate. The term is, of course, used in everyday parlance. We might well refer to someone as having reflective tendencies – meaning probably that s/he is somewhat thoughtful and contemplative and tends to muse over the meaning of experiences or perhaps some particular striking event.

This meaning is captured rather more formally in the comments made by Boud and colleagues in their book *Reflection: Turning Experience into Learning*.[2] They view reflection as a deliberate, purposeful, goal-directed activity through which the learner examines the meaning of the experience which s/he has undergone. The important difference from everyday reflection, which perhaps just happens, is that they are proposing that reflection should, be an important part of at least some learning situations. In these situations particular experiences can be 'set up' to prompt or stimulate such learning and encourage the learner to practise deliberate and planned reflection.

Communication and Group Behaviour was an optional unit within the independent study degree. It was a part of the skills focused set of units mentioned previously. The general outline of the unit had already existed when I arrived at Crewe+Alsager college. I am sure that at that early stage in my career I would have been nervous, even sceptical, about coming up with any course unit of this kind. However, since it was there I had to get on and think about how to teach it.

So, what was the nature and rationale of this unit? The basic aim was to use relevant aspects of social psychology to enable students to achieve a better appreciation of interpersonal interaction and group processes. So far, so good – this appears reasonably conventional and acceptable. However the further purpose of the unit was to enable students to improve their capacity to practise effectively in these contexts. Thus, the intention was that group members would, in various ways, achieve greater skill, become more competent operators in interpersonal and group contexts, and in so doing achieve a better understanding of themselves and the influence they had in these situations.

It was quite clear that if we were to achieve these aims, this could not be a conventionally taught academic unit. It took some time – a few years – to arrive at the best format and practice for the unit. Initially, I was fortunate to work with another tutor who was a qualified counsellor. This helped to 'free up' my ideas about what was acceptable and suitable practice in this context. In conjunction with my own more academic orientation, this allowed the development of an approach that combined academic content with opportunities for students to achieve a stronger awareness of their own social and personal experience.

What kind of teaching situation did this produce? It did not involve any kind of formal, didactic lectures. Instead the framework was supportive and enabling in style with the intention of facilitating personal growth and self-understanding. There was, though, still a carefully organised and structured teaching approach which had four main components.

The central one of these was a set of experiential exercises, and students took part in (or observed) one such exercise in each session of the unit. One exercise was where students were divided into two groups to participate in a problem solving task. One group received instructions which would incline them towards a co-operative stance. The other group was 'steered' towards being competitive.

The second component of the session was an immediate 'debriefing' discussion in which participants, and observers, would review the exercise experience. Students then had to complete reading which reviewed relevant research and theory. The final component of the teaching took place in the following week of the unit. This involved further discussion in which students reviewed the exercise experience again, but now in the light of the academic reading which they had completed over the previous week.

This kind of teaching set up is rather less predictable than a traditional lecture and follow up class. However, that open-endedness can add interest and excitement for both students and tutor. Exercises didn't always work quite as expected. Students didn't always do the reading they were supposed to. Nevertheless, I would say that the classes for the unit had a sense of involvement that could sometimes be lacking in more traditional units. The unit was always a popular one and student feedback was positive and enthusiastic.

One essential feature of any academic course unit which I have not touched on so far is that of assessment. What kind of assessed work would be appropriate for a relatively unconventional unit such as

Communication and Group Behaviour? Traditional essays or exams would not really be suitable. In keeping with the aims of the unit some task that required students to reflect further on their experiences of and reactions to the exercises used within the unit seemed appropriate.

After some trials and experimentation I developed a three way strategy. Firstly students kept a brief journal record of all the exercises in which they participated, assessed on a pass/fail basis only. Secondly, they were asked to write up three exercises, selected from the different parts of the course, in much greater detail. They needed to review their personal experience of the exercise, reflect on what they had learnt about themselves and their behaviour, and then link their exercise experience to relevant academic content.

The final component of the assessment was a reflective review of personal learning through the unit, completed at its end. In this review students were expected to discuss analytically and reflectively what they had learned about themselves and their own behaviour, feelings and interactional responses from the experience of the unit, and in the context of relevant theory.

Inevitably, reviews were influenced by the fact that they were part of the assessment process. Nevertheless, the comments and reflection produced by many of the students convinced me that important personal learning had, indeed, taken place. Just a very few excerpts from such reviews – both general and more specific – might give some sense of what students gained from the unit:[3]

> *The construction of the course is like a jig-saw, and the pieces fit together, intertwine and complement each other. They have helped me to develop a better understanding of the intricacies and problems that can arise from the mismanagement of oneself or a group. I have looked into myself as a result of this course unit and have found this very useful in knowing what my reactions are, or contemplating what they would be in a certain situation.*

During the whole unit of Communication and Group Behaviour, the class exercises have enabled me to understand many underlying aspects of everyday life that one takes for granted...Although the exercises were conducted in a somewhat unrealistic and constrained environment, they have nonetheless managed to increase personal awareness, better my communication skills, and have helped my self-confidence enormously.

In my daily life I am often outspoken and refuse to be ignored. I have never thought of myself as an aggressive person but maybe sometimes a little over enthusiastic. The work on assertiveness made me realise that when I want to express my opinion or my point of view I can come across in a very forceful and over zealous fashion.

During an exercise relating to deviance and cohesiveness I was really shocked at my attitude towards the deviants. I felt very angry at the intrusion of these latecomers. The group norms had already been established and I excluded them from any discussion. Upon reflection I realise this could have had an adverse effect upon the group decision, insulating information, not allowing changes to take place and stifling creative thought.

In the 'life-line' exercise, my line appeared to reflect a broad, simplistic outlook on life, which contrasted quite markedly with my partner's. His line reflected meticulous attention to life's details. In the short term/long term goals exercise I again became aware of my 'macro' approach to life. My goals are imprecise and based upon broad notions and ideals...His future was something for which he has a detailed plan, and as such was something to which he was looking forward. However, I tend to live from day to day, my future by contrast is something that will 'happen to me' as I have not really planned it.

Working alongside the students who followed the unit over the years was a positive and interactive experience. What did I learn? Linking personal experience with psychological research evidence and theory was an important reflective aim within this unit. In supporting students in this process I developed a better appreciation of how useful it could be in aiding my own personal insight. This is an approach that would have been frowned upon in the past by academic psychologists, and probably still is by some.

To engage in such reflection is demanding and difficult, but my own experience convinces me that it can be beneficial. I probably reflect on myself and my experience in a different kind of way as a consequence of developing and teaching this course unit. As it has turned out I think that this reflective approach has been a constructive one for me as I have worked to cope with the problems posed by having MS.

Career Retrospective…

Fortunately I can look back on my career with a considerable degree of satisfaction. I have not achieved anything very remarkable in terms of career progression – but then that was not my objective. I have never had any burning ambition to achieve promotion for the sake of it. My reward was personal satisfaction and enjoyment, and the worthwhile impact on the students whom I taught.

The teaching that I have done in various areas of psychology has been interesting and of personal benefit. Teaching other people is, of course, one of the best ways of learning. My teaching over the years has inevitably concentrated in particular areas of the discipline of psychology. But one of the major advantages of teaching in the higher education context is that the discipline is always advancing. There are new aspects to keep up with.

As well as the teaching itself, interaction with colleagues was also an important satisfaction. Working closely with the core independent studies team was an essential part of this, but the team expanded to include tutors from the youth and community and special needs area, and later newly appointed tutors in health studies. There was a real sense of enthusiasm and loyalty, feeling that we were doing something important and different.

Beyond this there were links with the humanities area and that of sports sciences. Tutors in these areas were also appointed to support the expansion taking place at the college in the second half of the nineteen seventies. It was an exciting time for everyone and provided a context for the development of social contact and friendship.

Undoubtedly, some of the greatest satisfaction in my career has come from my involvement with our degree by independent study. It was exciting to be taking a major part in this kind of innovative programme. There was also the continuing challenge of developing new teaching approaches and strategies which worked effectively in this different kind of teaching context. Part of the reward of this form of teaching was the opportunity to work closely with individual students in the supervision of their projects. These were often of considerable interest and took me into problem areas and academic literature that I might otherwise not have explored.

Now, I am also looking back on my career from the perspective of someone who has become disabled and developed a chronic illness. Coincidentally, some of the areas of psychology which I have taught have been ones which have a relevance for the coping process. My involvement with the processes and practice of reflective learning has been of particular benefit.

In addition the whole experience of having worked on our independent study degree provided a different perspective on coping. Especially early on it was useful to view the challenge of finding ways to live with MS as a particular kind of independent project. As with the projects completed by many students it had both practical and academic aspects. It was also something that I had to work at, take control of, and have responsibility for. It helped me to avoid considering myself as some kind of victim.

Notes and References

1. These quotations are taken from unpublished student feedback questionnaires.

2. Boud, D., Keogh, R. & Walker, D. (1985). *Reflection: Turning Experience into Learning*. London: Kogan Page.

3. The following quotations are taken from reflective reviews produced by students following the Communication and Group Behaviour course unit. These student comments have previously been published in Cuthbert, K. (1993). "Records of achievement in relation to personal learning," pp 102-103. In A. Assiter & E. Shaw (Eds), *Records of Achievement in Higher Education*, London: Kogan Page, The article provides a commentary on, and rationale for the assessment procedures adopted within the unit.

Chapter Four

MS and My Experience Of It

Diagnosis and After...

When we returned from our escape to Durham I still hadn't received a definite diagnosis. I wanted – needed – to know for sure. Days passed and I hadn't had any contact from the hospital. Impatiently, I got in touch with the hospital myself and obtained an appointment with the registrar I had seen initially.

I received the definite diagnosis that I did have Multiple Sclerosis on September 7th 1993 – what I had expected, and therefore at this stage not a huge shock. There was some relief that it wasn't anything worse – most especially a brain tumour. In some ways the final diagnosis experience came as an anticlimax.

I don't remember everything about that fairly short conversation, but one of the registrar's comments that sticks in my mind. was that when you get MS in middle age, as I did, you can't expect any remissions – the disease just gets gradually worse! Another comment was not to waste money on taking Evening Primrose oil supplements as they didn't do any good; in my view a remarkably unhelpful judgement. Maybe the evidence is not that precise, but Evening Primrose capsules are not particularly expensive, so even if there was only a small chance that they had some value they seemed to me to be worth taking.

I did accept another of the registrar's recommendations, to come in to the neurology ward as soon as possible and have a course of steroids (methyl prednesone) given intravenously. This is the most common treatment for an MS relapse. The steroids have an anti inflammatory effect. The usual judgement about their effectiveness is that they can reduce the length of a relapse, but otherwise are unlikely to influence the course of the disease.

Steroids can have serious side effects. At that point, immediately after my diagnosis, I didn't know much about them, so I thought it sensible to follow the medical recommendation. It wasn't any great joy to be back in hospital, which clearly reminded me that I was ill. The three day treatment period passed very quickly and I didn't experience any side effects, but there didn't appear to be any effect on my MS symptoms either.

With the new academic year about to start, the most pressing decision was could I start teaching again? Before the students returned I was involved in making a staff development presentation to other tutors. I completed this session, but it felt rather hard going from the physical/mobility point of view. I certainly couldn't move around easily in the classroom as previously taken for granted. After the session I went across to the refectory with some colleagues, and was very conscious of only being able to walk exceedingly slowly, with my companions having to adjust to my slower pace. It was as though I had got old very quickly and very suddenly. Although the staff development session had gone well and I was pleased about that, at the same time I still felt daunted and discouraged.

Though not keen to cause disruption and extra work for my colleagues, I decided that some time for rest, and hopefully recuperation, and some space for mental adjustment to changed circumstances was essential for my welfare. I was signed off sick by my GP. For the first time in my life I was 'off work' for a sustained period, and I didn't quite know when I would be going back.

I felt strange, and as though I was 'in limbo'. Clearly I was ill, but not in quite the usual way. I didn't have a temperature and I wasn't feverish; I wasn't sick in the sense of 'throwing up'; I wasn't in any kind of pain. There was no requirement to stay in bed. Susan Sontag has used the metaphor of 'entering the kingdom of the unwell' to refer to the experience of chronic illness.[1] It felt more akin to straddling the two worlds. I could still (with a walking stick for support) get out and take a short walk. If I could do this was I really ill and justified in being at home?

The ambiguity increased as I was still actually doing some university work. An academic can 'take work home'. Conveniently, I only lived half a mile or so from the college campus, so colleagues and students could easily come and visit. It would be difficult to find new supervisors for the three third year students whose independent projects I was supervising. We agreed that they would come to me, and I would hold supervisory meetings at home. Colleagues also came for a few administrative and planning meetings. I continued the writing of an academic paper, already accepted for presentation at an international conference.

Alongside this continuation of at least some aspects of my previous life I was trying hard to come to terms with the changes and uncertainty I faced. On many occasions during this period tears just overwhelmed me – I cried in a way that I had never done before. I was grieving for what I had lost – the comfort and security of my previous life, the things that I was used to doing, but could now no longer do.

There was a sense of disruption. Apart from grieving – which felt appropriate and altogether justified – what could I do? I took some comfort from other people's reactions to, and ways of dealing with, such threats. In my teaching of the course unit 'Communication and Group Behaviour' we had had some discussion of issues of identity. I had used an Open University audio tape titled 'Threats to Identity', that included comments from three people who had experienced such threat in different kinds of ways.

The first commentary was from Anthony Grey. He was one of the first political hostages to be captured and kept in isolation for a substantial period of time. He was detained during the middle 1960s by the Chinese Red Guards and kept a prisoner for a period of two years. A published account of his imprisonment is called *Hostage in Peking*.[2]

It perhaps seems rather melodramatic to compare my experience with his. I was not isolated, indeed I had loving support from my husband, friends and family. However, there were some common aspects; I was facing sudden change in the circumstances of my life and a considerable degree of uncertainty about the future. What impressed me most was Grey's determination to survive psychologically and motivationally; and keep intact his sense of himself. I resolved to adopt for myself some of that determination.

The other two commentators shared a closer similarity with my experience. Both had faced sudden onset of physical disability, but they had reacted in rather different ways. A woman became paralysed as a result of an accident. She described her son coming to visit her in hospital. As he walked into the ward she noticed his rather dishevelled appearance with tie at 'half mast'. This was perhaps not that unusual for a teenage boy, but her reaction was to see him as a 'motherless son', and she went on to imply that it might be better if he really was motherless – and she had been killed rather than severely injured.

The man was injured in a different kind of way, and in quite different circumstances. He had been shot at point blank range by a robber on the run from the police. This particular case had personal memories for me. The shooting had taken place at a cross-roads next to the river Dyfi, about twenty miles from Aberystwyth. The shooting had made the headlines of the local newspapers, as well as attracting some national coverage.

As a consequence of the shooting the then quite young policeman lost his sight completely. The commentary on the tape demonstrated an amazing lack of bitterness or anger. Anger was clearly justified especially since his blinding was not an accident but instead a consequence of something that somebody else had done to him.

Later in the tape there was a commentary on a climb up Snowdon. This is hardly an expedition I would have expected a blind man to undertake, let alone enjoy. However, he clearly did enjoy it; he took pleasure in being out in the open, physically active, feeling the wind on his face and noticing different sounds and smells. When I first heard the tape I had been impressed by his continuing delight in the natural world, and now it had a real personal resonance.

A relatively short tape can only give a 'snapshot' of someone's overall adjustment, but the strong impression was of someone who was at peace with himself and his world. This contrasted with the paralysed woman who had not fully accepted her condition. I cannot be sure that this is a wholly fair judgement. I do not know, for example, how long it had been since her accident. However, the tape brings it home how differently people can react to adversity. I knew that, as best I could, I needed to try to cultivate the acceptance of the blinded policeman, and the determination to achieve self survival of Anthony Grey.

As time went on during that autumn of 1993 I was aware that things were gradually improving. But there were some continuing strange bodily sensations. I still had the feeling of 'heavy legs' which had begun at the hotel in Berchtesgarten. Oddly though, they now came every other day with amazing regularity. I also often had a sensation of a tight band around my waist.

A kind of tightness also affected my feet, a feeling my shoes were too small for me although I knew perfectly well that they weren't. There was a degree of reduced sensation in my feet. The extent of this came home to me at the end of a trip to the local swimming pool. After changing back into my clothes I couldn't find my watch. I was fairly confident that I had put it safely somewhere, but as someone was giving me a lift home I had to hurry from the changing room and get quickly out to the car. At the other end I walked into the house. After a little bit of walking around at home I began to feel that there was something a little odder than usual about one of my feet although it wasn't a particularly strong sensation. I took my shoe off – and there was my missing watch!

However, in spite of such peculiarities, the general tendency was one of improvement. I could walk better. I took my stick out with me, but then didn't use it all the time – only at more difficult spots such as stepping off a kerb. I also found I was able to gradually increase the distances I walked, and was getting up the stairs more easily. So towards the end of that term, I considered whether I could manage the challenge of going back to work.

The Nature of MS...

As well as keeping up with some academic work, a major preoccupation during this early period of my MS was finding out more about this disease. To begin with I knew very little. The information I had prior to my own personal encounter with MS was limited and almost contradictory.

One of my sources of information was a fund-raising press campaign run by the MS Society at the end of the 1980s, the objective of the campaign obviously to increase donations to the society from the public. With this in mind it presented a stark and negative image of MS. The pictures were of beautiful young people with strips torn out of the image – across the eyes, or down the back – to represent the devastating effects of having MS. The presentation was one of helplessness and dependence.

Looking back from 2000 the MS Society's Marketing Director, Ken

Walker, commented that 'From an advertising point of view it was a great success and showered with accolades and awards'. From the perspective of 2000, however, the society admitted that the high impact was at considerable cost. The campaign had been upsetting to many people with MS, especially the newly diagnosed.[3]

I saw this advertising campaign before I had MS, and before I knew anything very much about it. It certainly caught my attention, but with the result that it made me quite angry. As a psychologist interested in self processes, I felt that the campaign was in many ways unethical. For people recently diagnosed with MS it would be likely to disrupt their confidence in their capability to continue managing their own lives.

Fortunately, as someone who now did have MS, I possessed some different information to counter balance the images provided in this campaign. During the Easter of 1991 Pete and I had visited my sister and brother-in-law and their family who live in Boston in the U.S. While we were there the *Boston Globe* newspaper ran a feature on the Boston marathon, and one article reviewed the training and performance of a lady with MS who was running the marathon. She had done so successfully, and reported that she had actually beaten her husband! So, fortunately, I knew that having MS didn't always lead to complete helplessness. But I really needed to know more than this – so my personal MS research campaign had started.

A book that I discovered early on after my diagnosis became a useful source of information, but more importantly, a source also of positive encouragement. As I soon discovered, many books and articles on MS emphasise either directly, or implicitly, the likelihood and probably the inevitability of physical decline. The book by Judy Graham, entitled *Multiple Sclerosis: A self help guide to its management* certainly does not 'fudge' the seriousness of the disease. However, its tone is positive and encouraging. Its greatest value is an emphasises on what a person with MS can do for themselves with the goal of maintaining positive health, and taking charge of the illness experience. Reading this book led to my taking care over my diet – especially avoiding saturated fats as much as possible, and confirmed the importance of exercise.[4]

But what is possible? What is the nature of this disease? The first thing to be said is that its causation is certainly highly complex, and probably more complex than anyone yet understands. The account offered here can only hint at some of this complexity.

Multiple sclerosis is both an auto-immune and a neurological disease.[5] Our immune systems normally enable our bodies to resist and overcome infection. However, in a number of diseases, and MS is one of these, the immune system turns to attacking systems within the person's body, rather than outside invaders. These are the auto-immune diseases. Rheumatoid arthritis is another well-known example.

The particular bodily system which comes under attack in MS is the central nervous system, which underlies the neurological character of the disease. Somehow the normal blood-brain barrier is breached. As a consequence, areas of inflammation develop within the central nervous system. The crucial consequence of this inflammation is that there is breakdown of myelin within the nervous tissue. Myelin is a fatty material which provides a sheath around the fibres of nerve cells which have a crucial function in transmitting messages within our nervous systems. If there is loss of myelin, the transmission of these nerve impulses and messages becomes less efficient.

Inflammation can decline over time. Also, there is now evidence that it is possible for myelin to regenerate, although neurologists do not yet understand the circumstances in which this happens. Thus, damage is not necessarily final and absolute. However, as the disease progresses it is also the case that hard plaques, or scars of damage are likely to form in areas of demyelination. This kind of damage represents the sclerosis of the disease name, and it is multiple because the damage occurs, to a greater or lesser degree, through the central nervous system.

Perhaps it is becoming evident how MS can be quite a varied disease. Symptoms derive from the interruption to the functioning of the neurones within the central nervous system. But the extent of the problem will depend on how much demyelination and plaque formation occurs, and where, within the brain and central nervous system, it happens.

Scientists who research into MS have done their best to describe and classify these varying patterns. At its simplest two main categories are proposed. In the most common relapse–remission form of the disease periods of worsening symptoms are interspersed with periods of remission in which recovery may be pretty well complete, or more partial. In the other main form, chronic progressive MS, there are less likely to be definable relapses, and it is more a case of symptoms and disability gradually accumulating and increasing.

However, the simplicity of this two-way classification is really very much an over-simplification which hides a much more complex reality. Each of the two forms shades into various sub-types. In many ways it is perhaps more appropriate (if more confusing) to think of a spectrum of categories and symptoms.

The relapse-remission form of MS can itself be highly variable since the relapses may be of varying severity, come at varying time intervals, and the recovery between the relapses may be to varying degrees. The most fortunate have a benign form of the disease with perhaps one or two relapses, but with pretty well full recovery, and then apparently no further experience of the disease. At the other end of this range other individuals don't make a good recovery from their ongoing relapses, and so increasing disability is cumulative. This form of the disease has been labelled by some commentators as 'chronic relapsing progressive MS'.

The chronic progressive form of the disease which is progressive in an ongoing way (that is without discernible remission) is categorised as either primary or secondary progressive. The primary progressive form is progressive from the start, and in a minority of cases can be severely so, leading quite early on to severe disability. More commonly secondary progressive MS follows on from an earlier relapse–remission stage. It is often suggested that this kind of progression is the eventual fate of everyone who has MS.

However, it is important to emphasise that the whole classification of symptoms and forms of MS is a descriptive one. There is no causative model associated with this attempted summary of symptoms and their progression. Thus the categorisation does not lead to any reliable prediction of what will happen for any individual with MS. There are too many exceptions to the suggested patterns and there is, as yet, no adequate understanding of why the disease progresses in any particular way. The best that seems to be offered in the prediction line is that what has happened in the first five years (or maybe ten) of having had the disease may give some kind of rough guide to the future. So, from the perspective of the person who actually has MS, one of the clearest features of the disease has to be the high degree of uncertainty which it involves.

Ideally, we would all like a cure, but, that is probably some way off. Progress is certainly being made, and there are now drugs that reduce the frequency of relapses in the relapse-remission form of the disease. It is also important that symptom management treatments are improving considerably. At the same time, it is always the case that drug treatments have side effects. It can be difficult to balance improvements in symptoms against unpleasant side effects. Uncertainty continues, and decision making is not always easy. There are psychological challenges in adjusting to illness, but these can also be present in deciding about treatments.

Back to Work – and Play…

So how were things going for me? Fortunately there was positive progress. Towards the end of November 1993 it was clear matters had improved considerably. I could move around more easily both inside and outside the house. Though I always took my stick with me when I went outside, it was for security rather than necessity. Despite what the registrar had said at diagnosis in September, it was pretty obvious that I was moving into a remission.

Of course, I still had MS but I was beginning to adjust so I needed to get back to at least a degree of normality. That meant returning to my teaching role, and I decided to try working for the last few weeks of that Autumn term. I didn't do a full timetable and obviously we were coming up to the Christmas vacation so it was a helpfully gentle way back.

I have always felt just a slight degree of apprehension when starting teaching again after a gap – usually the student summer vacation period. Now, I had been away from it all for pretty well six months, if I included the examination period of the previous June. But everything went better than I could have hoped. I was welcomed back by my students who expressed their concern for my welfare. I soon overcame that slight degree of nervousness; the teaching went OK – I hadn't forgotten how to do it!

So that Christmas we celebrated! We were not just enjoying the festive season, there was also celebration of getting back to something approaching ordinary life. We had our usual kind of Christmas with my parents and sister in Aberystwyth, but we relished the ordinary things in a very special kind of way.

The following term continued to go well. I was soon re-involved in the whole business of teaching, and planning for the future on our independent study degree. In fact, in this respect, it was quite an exciting time. With a couple of colleagues I was planning a new first year course unit. This developed further the kind of support we gave to first year students in preparation for their later independent study. We would begin teaching the unit in the following September.

Gradually over the Spring of 1994 I was able to extend the distance I could walk. Pete and I took advantage of this with short walks in the local countryside at the weekends. I also got back to swimming, indeed I did more than I had for some years. Conveniently there was a local leisure centre swimming pool across the road from the university and I made sure that I took time for regular lunch time swims.

As February turned into March we felt that we needed more than just weekend outings. We wanted a holiday to enjoy, to recuperate from the stress and strain of the past months, and to celebrate the improvements in my health and capability. It is not that easy to take a holiday during university term time, but we both managed to negotiate a week during the May examination period.

After some discussion we decided that the Swiss Bernese Oberland would make a good destination, to be back in the mountains, and Switzerland would have plenty of the most impressive kind. Still not being able to take long hikes on foot we needed other ways of getting into and up the mountains. In this respect we knew that Switzerland would be ideal because of the excellent availability of access by cog railways, chair lifts and gondolas.

It was a wonderful holiday in the village of Wilderswill, just outside Interlaken, with easy railway access up to Grindlewald and Wengen, and it was fantastic to have such a good stay amidst this marvellous and impressive scenery. We really enjoyed being up in the mountains, and especially pleased that I could manage a couple of longer and more demanding walks, more than I had thought possible. It felt like a major triumph!

As 1994 progressed into 1995 I settled back into the usual routine of academic work and teaching, but also with some new departures. We found the planning, and then the implementation, of our new unit on supporting students in managing their own learning both challenging and interesting. I had also decided, rather late in my career, to use my research into student learning within the independent study degree, to register for a PhD. So my working life was pretty busy. I could never forget that I had MS – there were always underlying reminders – but in most ways life was back to normal.

In physical terms I was doing pretty well. I was mostly walking without a stick. During the Easter of 1995 we decided to try a holiday in the lake District with the intention of doing as much walking as I could manage. Everything about that week exceeded our best hopes. We booked rather at the last minute, but found a comfortable guest house on the outskirts of Grasmere. The weather was kind to us and again I was able to walk further than I expected, and over reasonably demanding terrain. We walked distances of up to seven miles on successive days and climbed some of the minor tops around Grasmere. It was splendid to be really, properly out in the hills again.

I was feeling that if I was lucky and my MS could stay like this it wouldn't be too bad, and the disruption to my life would be minimal. At the same time I knew very well that there was absolutely no guarantee that my good fortune would be maintained.

MS as a Chronic Illness…

Clearly multiple sclerosis is a chronic illness. Its essential feature is that it doesn't get better. Currently there is no cure. When I first got MS the other chronic diseases of which I was immediately aware were rheumatoid arthritis and Parkinson's disease. They were both clearly progressive like MS and were potentially quite severely disabling. Rheumatoid arthritis shares with MS a frequent onset in early adulthood and it is also an auto-immune disease. Parkinson's disease, like MS, has a neurological basis, but usually with a later onset.

Unfortunately, despite the progress of modern medicine, there are still many other diseases out there not easily curable. There might be some debate over a definitive list but obvious and well-known contenders for inclusion are late onset diabetes, osteo-arthritis, asthma and Aids. Many would also include heart disease, stroke and some forms of cancer. Some of these diseases are associated with the ageing process, and therefore become more salient in a society in which general improvements in health care enable many of us to live longer.

To what extent do these various illnesses have things in common? In terms of the medical challenge posed, both to medical caregivers, and to the person with the disease there are crucial differences. However, from a psychological perspective, there is much in common; there is a psychological as well as a physical challenge. Although in MS (and other diseases) it is certainly the case that treatment of symptoms (e.g. tremor, muscular spasms) has improved, nevertheless, in this chronic illness situation psychological coping is, in many ways, as important as medical management.

Health psychologists have suggested some important ways in which chronic illness differs from acute illness – that is the kind of illness from which one is expected to recover.[6] The most important point is implicit in this comment. Chronic illness is, by its nature, long lasting – full recovery is not expected. Having such a disease means that life changes and a degree of acceptance and adjustment is required.

A further point, already emphasised in relation to MS and which is characteristic of many other chronic illnesses, is a degree of ongoing uncertainty. Symptoms may change – either intensifying, or fading away, on a day to day, week to week, or longer term basis. Also, nobody ever knows how bad it will get. Will one become severely incapacitated, or be just mildly affected? Such uncertainty is disturbing and stressful.

Another area of ambiguity concerns the extent or sense in which one is really ill. Unlike someone with a moderate or severe short term illness, or other medical problem, the individual with a chronic illness would not generally take to their bed. Most likely they will not attract quite the kind of care, attention and sympathy normally devoted to someone who is temporally ill. In sociological terms the chronically ill do not continuously occupy the status of sick people. For much of the time many chronically sick people will continue to participate, in the usual kind of way, in everyday life. We are both 'ill' and 'not ill' at the same time. This can create difficulties in terms of how far one pushes the role of being ill, or alternatively how strongly one resists it. There can also be problems for other people in terms of their having to make judgements about the extent to which they should treat us as being 'a bit ill', or just 'as normal'.

An important psychological challenge for many of us who develop a chronic illness is the degree of disruption in how we view ourselves – our sense of identity. There may be things, which used to be important, that we can no longer do. I cannot walk easily. Certainly I can no longer ski. It could become difficult to continue in employment, or look after a family as easily as in the past. Adjusting and accommodating to these changes is not an easy matter.

Progression…

For me, the next period of change in my MS arrived in the autumn of 1995. This time it didn't come suddenly – but instead rather insidiously. From that autumn I realised that when we were out walking my legs were getting tired more quickly than they had been. I had to start using my stick again, and even then began to experience loss of co-ordination in my left leg, at first after walking perhaps a couple of miles, but then after shorter distances. It was often a struggle to get back to our starting point. I had to stop and rest along the way.

After having had such a wonderful period of remission, during which time my life had almost got back to normal, I found it very upsetting and very discouraging to have things getting worse again. I had known it could happen at any time, but that knowledge didn't really help any when it did! Through the end of 1995, and into 1996, my physical capability declined quite considerably, and felt I was back where I had been in September 1993.

Once more I couldn't walk properly, or very far. I found it frustrating, exasperating and depressing, being back to needing to use a stick to walk everywhere apart from around the house. Before long it seemed the most sensible and safest procedure to use one indoors as well.

My balance was deteriorating beyond the level of my initial relapse. I began to have some quite dramatic falls. I knew that I was just about to fall, but there was nothing that I could do to save myself, and I would usually hit the floor with quite a crash. If Pete was anywhere in the house, he would come rushing to see what had happened.

Fortunately, and I am not quite sure how this was achieved, I never seriously hurt myself. (Just possibly it was lots of experience of falling down on skiing holidays!) Shocked, perhaps shaken and sometimes a bit bruised – but nothing more. If Pete was there, I would get some physical comforting. Otherwise, after a few minutes recovery time on the floor, I would begin to get up slowly, sit for a bit longer, and then get on with what I had been doing. Physically I could get up and get on, but I felt very upset by these falls, an indicator things were getting even worse than they had before.

Alongside these discouraging experiences, I was still looking out for any positive signs as we moved through the winter of 1996. I was hoping for, searching for any sign of the kind of improvement that had happened after my previous MS attack. Some days things seemed to be a bit better, I could move more easily, climb the stairs a little more readily, or maybe I'd take a short walk and not feel quite so tired. Then my hopes increased as it seemed that improvement was really coming. I would feel happy and positive, and want to celebrate.

Then, over the next few days, when the slight improvement didn't continue, my hopes would be dashed. It was not a real improvement.

Maybe things had improved a little temporarily – or maybe I had just thought they had. The emotional let-down afterwards was devastating – much worse than the physical shock of falling onto the floor. I wanted to curl up into a ball and shut out the external world. In spite of these awful negative reactions it was still very difficult not to hope when there seemed to be any kind of positive indication. I wanted so much for things to get better.

But the roller coaster of hope, then the loss of hope of any improvement was really very difficult to cope with. After a period of experiencing these ups and downs, I knew I had to stop myself hoping that a remission might be beginning. It was a hard thing to do – but the negative upset and huge disappointment afterwards was not worth the little bit of hope. If things really did improve, that would soon become evident over a period of weeks. It didn't happen, so I had to begin to reconcile myself to continuing disability.

It was at this point, in the spring of 1996, that I decided it was time to get back in touch with the neurology department at the local hospital. Through my GP I got an appointment with the consultant whom I had seen briefly after my diagnosis. In his judgement my MS had probably changed to become chronic progressive in form. He suggested that it was worth trying steroid treatment again – although he didn't hold out a great deal of hope that it would be greatly beneficial.

So, on June 21st 1996, I was back in hospital and had methyl prednesone steroid treatment over a three day period. Since this was my second experience I knew what to expect. Fortunately three days goes reasonably quickly so it was soon all over. Then it was just a case of waiting to see if any improvement materialised. Despite my earlier experience of trying to quench hope, and the consultant's pessimism, there were some lingering sparks of positive hope. But over the next few months nothing changed. My last chance of improvement seemed to have gone. Instead, the likelihood was of further physical decline. It was another time of tears and mourning.

Then there was a new and unexpected blow. I suddenly realised that when I had my right eye closed things were pretty fuzzy. I have worn glasses (or contact lenses) since I was a teenager, and my left eye is my best one. Now my sight in that eye had declined quite considerably. As well as the fuzziness, there were strange light effects – especially coloured rings around things.

Coming on top of my walking difficulties and the falling about the place, this added to the sense that things were just getting worse and worse. I knew that eyesight problems did happen in MS. These could be long term and people could be registered blind. Even when I was feeling really upset about not being able to walk properly, I would sometimes think that losing my sight would be the most difficult thing to cope with. How could I manage ? I just didn't want to think about it.

I had to do something! I saw my GP and got a hospital appointment for more steroid treatment. Generally there is a wait for these things. In the meantime my luck changed – to some extent. Fortunately, inflammation of the neural nerve, or optic neuritis, is something that in most cases does improve. After four or five weeks my sight began to improve, and soon it was a lot better. I didn't need the steroid treatment after all. It was a tremendous relief!

Cultivating Resilience...

My eyesight was better – but nothing else was showing any signs of improvement. How should...could I react to this chronic, progressive state of MS? For me this was a period of major mental readjustment. A degree of readjustment had been going on since I had had the MS diagnosis, but, I had also experienced a good period of remission when life had almost got back to normal. Now, though, the pressure was on to cope, manage and readjust.

What could I do? Perhaps trial and error exploration, or supportive discussion with others would help. But, as a psychologist the most obvious strategy was to investigate relevant psychological literature. The search through discussions of coping under pressure had a personal rather than an academic objective. Rather a dry and almost abstract form of readjustment, but identifying these strategies was important and aided my understanding of the challenging new personal world I was in. This was cognitive rather than physical readjustment. I had to work out the best ways of managing my changed life. When people inquired how I was doing I answered that physical activity was obviously limited, but I was doing a lot of cognitive work and readjustment.

As indicated, one of the most troubling aspects of having MS, or many other chronic illnesses, is the accompanying uncertainty. Uncertainties of various kinds mean that it is difficult to feel in control of one's life. Believing that you are reasonably in control is usually seen as a desirable state, both by the ordinary person, and for psychological adjustment. The idea of control, for psychologists, has come to be quite a complex one.[7]

At a personal level, if I believe that what I do, and how I manage my life has important consequences, then I am more likely to get out there, do things, and take action. This kind of belief is positive and adaptive. The less positive, more maladaptive situation is if I believe that I am at the mercy of fate or chance. In that case it will feel as though what I do has no real impact on the world. It is only a short step to feeling that it is not worth bothering to do anything.

It is probably clear why someone with MS (or other chronic illness) can easily be led into believing that they have limited control over their lives. So, the attitude might easily be why bother? The more adaptive position (though easier said than done) is to make appropriate and realistic distinctions between what can, and what cannot be controlled. For many chronic illnesses, and most probably for MS, the course of the illness itself cannot be changed, but some symptoms can be managed. Inability to make the appropriate differentiation can lead to considerable emotional distress as a result of effort to change the unchangeable.

A different aspect of dealing psychologically with difficulties in one's life is called benefit finding. This is really searching for the proverbial silver lining – trying to notice and identify any benefits which can emerge out of the difficult circumstances. Engaging in benefit finding 'predicts emotional and physical adaptation months and even years later'.[8] Even though much of my period off work was a very difficult time I was still able to enjoy the benefits of a more relaxed pace of life.

It is interesting that you don't have to find lots of benefits. Just having identified one seems to be sufficient to trigger a positive reaction. Perhaps it is more about frame of mind than anything else – a preparedness to accept and recognise that positive outcomes are possible. On the other hand, it is no help to have other people point out benefits to you, for that is likely to be seen as somebody trying to minimise the difficulties you are experiencing. Benefit finding, as so much in this adaptation process, has to be something that you do for yourself.

Another linked cognitive dimension receiving increased attention from psychologists in recent years is tending to have generally optimistic, or alternatively rather more pessimistic judgements about the future.[9] Is this relevant to coping with MS? Is it possible to be optimistic when one has a chronic disease? Well, maybe! A fair amount of the research into optimism and pessimism has been conducted in the context of coping with adverse circumstances, for example people dealing with coronary bypass surgery and failed in-vitro fertilisation.

In these kinds of circumstances, optimists are more likely to confront a problem 'head on' and not distance themselves from it. As a consequence they are more likely to take a problem solving approach.

They will make plans for how they are going to deal with the difficulties they face. Optimists tend to dwell less on the negative aspects which helps to avoid distress.

Pessimists, on the other hand, are more likely to engage in wishful thinking and do things that provide temporary distraction, but do not help to solve the problem. In the most difficult and uncontrollable situations, optimists face the reality of the situation, rather than denying it. If one cannot always be optimistic that things will turn out well then perhaps there is an important value in accepting things as they are. The idea of acceptance can easily be seen in a negative light – as a form of fatalistic resignation. But maybe there is a different way of thinking about acceptance.

I have found the idea of a positive 'take' on acceptance to be a very useful and encouraging one. Faced with a chronic illness, some difficult things just have to be accepted. But to be able to see that acceptance as providing a basis for moving forward is very helpful.

The two psychologists who have made the major contribution to this work on pessimism and optimism, but also acceptance, are Charles Carver and Michael Scheier. They have commented that:

> ...denial... means attempting to hold onto a world view that is no longer valid. In contrast, acceptance implies a restructuring of one's experience so as to come to grips with the reality of one's situation...The acceptance we have in mind is a willingness to admit that a problem exists, or that an event has happened – even an event that may irrevocably alter the fabric of the person's life. We are not talking, however, about a stoic resignation, a fatalistic acceptance of the negative consequences to which the problem or event might lead.[10]

All these strategies have in common that they are facing problems in a positive kind of way. They involve searching out solutions. But, it is not sensible to always focus on problems. There are times when diversions from the problems posed by having a chronic illness are necessary and beneficial.

Notes and References

1. Sontag, S. (1977). *Illness as Metaphor*. New York: Doubleday Anchor

2. Grey, A. (1970). *Hostage in Peking*. London: Pan Books.

3. Receiving the message loud and clear. An article on charity advertising in MS Matters, Sep/Oct, 2000.

4. Graham. J. (1992). *Multiple Sclerosis: The Self-help Guide to its Management*. London: Thorsons.

5. My account on the nature of MS draws on articles which have been published in MS Matters and a number of guides to the disease e.g. Benz, C. (1988). *Coping with Multiple Sclerosis*. London: Optima.
Sibley, W.A. (1996). *Theraputic Claims in Multiple Sclerosis*. New York: Demos.

6. See, for example the discussion of chronic illness in chapter 7 of Radley, A. (1994). *Making Sense of Illness*. London: Sage.

7. The idea of control, or more specifically locus of control has been an important one in the study of personality. Introductory discussions are provided in many text books on personality. A good one is in Hampson, S.E. (1988) (2nd Ed.). *The Construction of Personality: An introduction*. London: Routledge.

8. Tennen, H. & Affleck, G. (2002). Benefit-finding and benefit-reminding. In C.R. Snyder & S.L. Lopez (Eds), *Handbook of Positive Psychology*. New York: Oxford University Press.

9. There is a good, but quite demanding discussion of optimism versus pessimism in Carver, C.S. & Scheier, M.F. (2002). "Optimism." In C.R. Snyder & S.L. Lopez (Eds), *Handbook of Positive Psychology, pp. 231-234*. New York: Oxford University Press.

10. This quotation is taken from p. 237 within the above article.

Chapter Five

Distraction: *Our* 'Grand Design'

A Long-Term Plan...

Kevin McCloud's *Grand Design* television series on Channel 4 has now publicised the possibilities – and the pleasures and pains – of self build to a wide audience. Pete and I first thought about a self build back in the early eighties. This kind of project obviously has to be a joint thing in a fundamental kind of way. However, in our case, it is also true to say that Pete has been the prime mover. We have both had a long term interest in issues of conservation and 'preserving the planet'. For Pete this led to an interest in energy efficient and autonomous housing design. He acquired a substantial collection of relevant books which I found interesting too – at least the less technical aspects.

Pete was, and is, interested in the technical side as well. Although ending up as an academic, Pete has always had practical interests – and the skills and capabilities to go with these interests. He enjoys making and building things. As a teenager he built himself not just one, but three sailing dinghies. Also, with his father, he installed a generator and electrical system at their rather isolated North Devon home, which was not connected to mains electricity.

Since we got together there have been various other projects, early on some items of furniture; later, a more ambitious project was constructing a solar hot water system from old radiators and such like in the first house we owned. Then there was the car – a kit car which was an MG look alike – a rather smart job with a lovely cream body work finish, beige imitation leather hood and traditional bucket type seats.

In our early sortie into self build we got as far as just beginning to look around for building plots. But we didn't come across anything which was really desirable and other projects and events intervened. We bought ourselves a new house – but one built by developers on a small estate. We abandoned the project for the time-being.

An Ideal Plot…

At the beginning of the nineties Pete suggested we should reconsider self-build possibilities. We bought more books, took out a subscription to the monthly magazine 'Build It' and began to collect and file information about processes and products. We also bought a couple of books of house plans to enable us to think about designs and lay-out for our ideal house.

We also visited actual buildings. We revisited the Centre for Alternative Technology just north of Machynlleth. We had a day out at Milton Keynes in order to see a set of about half a dozen innovative, and environmentally friendly houses which were available for viewing, later to be sold off to private purchasers. We also visited more traditional show houses on various local developments in order to get a different kind of perspective on how various designs would appear and feel in built form. Another information collecting foray was to the Building Centre in London. My strongest memory from there was the huge display of varieties of bricks in a multitude of different colours and textures.

Essential for any self build project is first to find a building plot, quite a difficult matter. The usual way of getting information is through estate agents, who sell plots as well as houses, though only a limited number of building plots come onto the market. Single plots for self-build purposes are often where a householder with a large garden sells off a part as an infill building plot. Our first strategy was obviously to investigate local estate agents, and then leave information about our requirements so that they could contact us if anything suitable came onto their books. However, before any of the agents had time to contact us, we found a plot completely by chance.

I had cycled over to the next town, Sandbach, which was about five miles away from our home in Alsager. (This was in the time before MS.) On my way home and on the outskirts of the town, I happened to glance down a side road: at the end of the road I could just see a For Sale notice. I don't know what it was that persuaded me to take a closer look, but I did. To my amazement I discovered a plot rather than a house that was being advertised. This first quick inspection suggested a degree of promise. It was a reasonably sized corner plot and I could see across the road the houses finished and there were views of fields and countryside. I rode home in a state of considerable excitement.

Further examination of the plot itself and of the information from the estate agent (the relevant agent had offices in the next town, and not one we had contacted) confirmed my earlier positive perceptions. The plot had initial outline planning permission for a detached dwelling, positioned on the edge of the green belt on the outskirts of town. Just beyond the road became a single track, but still tarmacked, lane with fields on either side.

Discovering there were other purchasers seriously interested, we would need to move quickly if we wished to secure the plot, and, fortunately, this was possible. We do not usually take such important decisions quite so quickly, but couldn't imagine finding a better plot. Moving fast was, in this case, a necessary decision, so late in 1990 we became the proud owners of an empty building plot.

First Design...

So, we had got our plot – sooner than we thought, and we needed to start planning for something to go on it. Fortunately, unlike many self-builders, we hadn't had to borrow money to buy the plot, and hence weren't under major pressure to get on as fast as possible with the plans, and then the build. But, we still wanted to progress.

First, we had to get serious over the design, easier now we knew the size and shape of the plot onto which the house would have to fit. We started work on sketching out possible arrangements. After a few trials, modifications, and a deal of mulling over how things might work for practical living, we had an initial design that we felt reasonably satisfied with. Surprisingly, mine was the greater influence on the design. I say surprisingly because Pete thinks more readily in three dimensions than I.

The second requirement was starting to think about the building process. An important first decision was whether it should be a traditional build, often referred to as bricks and blocks, or timber framed. We favoured the latter from early on because of better insulation levels.

A further decision was about the management and organisation of the build – who would do it. Self-build doesn't mean, or doesn't require, actually doing the work yourselves. Some intrepid souls do, of course, do it all. But most self-builders get professional builders to do at least the greater part of the work. Ideally, Pete would have liked to have made a reasonable 'hands on' contribution to the build. However, realistically, with both of us working full-time in quite demanding jobs, this didn't seem a sensible option.

Our first step in getting the professionals in was to contact a national firm who specialised in doing the design work and producing the timber frame for customer's builds. As part of the package they would use the firm's architects to produce professional plans and then apply for detailed planning permission. It took us a while to get our design fully worked out, but eventually we were at the stage of having detailed plans prepared.

The next task would be to get detailed planning permission for our design. Since we were on the spot and the build firm we were using was some distance away, it seemed sensible for us to make the initial informal contact with the planning authorities. We made our first visit to the planning office, and soon found that things were not going to be quite as straightforward as we hoped.

In the planning officer's opinion, our intended new house was going to be too large and imposing, especially in the context of being next to a pair of Victorian cottages. We were a bit surprised at this objection. The house – a reasonably compact four bedroomed detached – would not be that large. We had chosen bricks, roof tiles and an exterior design compatible with next door in particular. Also the whole road had a mixture of housing styles, this being one of the things which had appealed to us. There were thirties semis across the road, fifties dormer bungalows immediately around the corner, and a few larger detached houses down the road.

However, it is best to have the planning officer on your side when the formal application goes forward, so we decided to work on persuasion. Pete took lots of photographs of the site and surrounding houses. He then drew up some excellent pictures, from a number of viewpoints, of how things would look with our house in position. Later discussion with the planning officer suggested that we were getting somewhere with our persuasion campaign. But then problems began to appear from quite a different quarter.

High Court Involvement…

Most commentaries on self-build say that there will be problems of one kind or another sometime in the build, but we met our first serious problems before we'd even started building! The first indication came when the representative of the timber frame company with whom we had worked phoned us up to break the news that he had been sacked. Clearly he was upset, as were we, because we had had a good working relationship with him.

After that our relationship with the company went downhill rapidly. They didn't keep us informed about what was going on, but were pressing ahead with the application for planning permission. They did let us know when that was turned down. We were surprised because we had thought by that time that we had the planning officer on our side. Then, when we did get the full information we found that it was their incompetence that had caused the problem. The planning application they had made had not conformed to the basic regulations about space around buildings – that is between the proposed house and the boundaries of the plot.

They still sent us a bill. We refused to pay – or at least the part that related to the failed planning application. They took out a summons against us to get payment. Since the amount of money involved was relatively small, and below the limit for the Small Claims Court, Pete mistakenly set up our defence through this mechanism. Unbeknown to us the building company was actually taking proceedings through the High Court, so the appearance there was that we had failed to provide any defence.

The first thing we knew about the problem was when a letter came to say that judgement had been made against us and we must pay the money within a short space of time. If we didn't the bailiffs would be around to confiscate effects to cover the money owed! In our secure middle class life nothing quite like this had previously loomed up in our lives. The drama of the event was accentuated by it happening immediately after I had come out of hospital after my first steroid treatment for MS in September 1993.

We obviously needed to act fast. Pete applied for a stay of execution on the judgement. The night before the hearing in front of a judge in the local court, the firm involved phoned us up. They had obviously now had second thoughts about the whole business, probably realising that they were not going to get their money quite as easily as they had thought! We, of course, intended to go through with the hearing so that we could get the judgement properly overturned.

The hearing turned out to be a much less auspicious occasion than I had expected. We met the judge in his rooms at the court. But nobody turned up to represent the firm who had taken action against us to recover the money. Clearly this didn't put them in a favourable light with the judge concerned. We went to a waiting room while he tried to make contact with the plaintiff's solicitors.

When we returned it was clear that the judge was very cross and his only concern was to 'tie up' the case in such a way that it would be impossible for the firm to try to extract the money from us in the future. He decided that the best procedure was to accept our petition and then throw the case out. For us, after a few very stressful days, it all ended happily. We didn't have to pay the money, nor did we have to pay any costs.

New Plans...

I suppose that we could, at this stage, have given up and aborted our plan to self-build. But it didn't seriously cross either of our minds to do so. We would need to move house anyway. Our then house didn't have a downstairs loo. Depending on what happened to my MS, which was of course unknown, that could become a necessity. So, we decided to proceed with our self-build intentions, but start the house planning process from scratch in order that we could take account of our changed circumstances.

We could have gone so far as to build a bungalow instead of a house, but neither of us were too keen on this idea. In any case, a bungalow wouldn't have fitted very well on the site we had. We decided instead to include a downstairs bedroom, bathroom, and study space for me, so that if absolutely necessary I could live on that floor.

Where should we start with the new plans? This time Pete took the lead in producing an outline plan. His inspiration came from a copyright free, 'salt box' design from one of his American books on autonomous housing. The essential feature of the design is that the living/kitchen/dining area is wholly open-plan, very beneficial if my mobility difficulties increased and, anyway, it just seemed interesting and attractive in itself. The other important feature is a cathedral ceiling, extending to the roof line, and with a pair of velux windows for extra light over the main living area. The stairs go up from the far end of the living area and lead to a gallery landing which overlooks the ground floor living area. Although in some ways it had been a wrench to abandon our initial plans, we began to feel rather excited by our new, more innovative, design.

Initially, Pete drew up a plan of our proposed design. (His O level in technical drawing has proved to be a very useful qualification!) Then we engaged an architect to polish these up for us and submit them for planning permission. Having had enough of dealing at something of a distance with a large, nationally based firm we selected a local architect recommended by the Association of Self Build Architects. Strangely enough, although his firm had offices nearby, he actually turned out to an American working in this country.

Our next task was to select a building firm who could do most of the work for us. Again, we tried to find a relatively local firm with whom we could have reliable personal contact and who had experience of timber frame construction. The self-build magazines carry advertisements and accounts of houses already built by builders who are in this market.

We made preliminary investigations into a number of firms, but then whittled this down to two main contenders. We discussed our plans with them, found out about their building experience, and viewed one or two of their completed builds. After our previous bad experience we were somewhat wary. We wanted people with whom we felt personally comfortable, and whom we could trust in the building of our house. This time we made sure that there was more personal contact, and more time to assess their building experience and competence.

Meanwhile, we were continuing to investigate and gather information about the whole building process – reading books, articles and informative publicity literature from the firms who manufacture, or deal in building components. Our reference files covered everything, bricks, roof tiles, window frames, insulation, plaster board, stairs, internal and external doors, and so on. One of the pleasures, although this can merge into pain and indecision, is that the self build option means you get to choose everything. On the more technical side, we (especially Pete) became experts in underfloor heating, mechanical ventilation and heat recovery systems and pipes for plumbing and various other things.

By the end of 1995 we had planning permission for our new design. We had also made our decision about which builders we would engage, choosing a family firm called Christian Torsten, based at Wem, in Shropshire. Unusually, the firm was headed by a woman, Marina Blank, together with her two sons Carl and Otto. The family also had a somewhat unusual history. They had lived in Sweden for quite a substantial period of time and, as a result, had become knowledgeable about the timber framed approach which is the dominant building technology in that country. Back in this country they established their own company producing timber frames for house building, then progressed to full house builds for clients who wanted that.

We had been unlucky to have the problem with our first building firm. In retrospect though, this turned out to be fortunate in that we hadn't started building prior to my MS diagnosis, and so could adapt our plans accordingly. Now, we were all ready to proceed with our new and better design in combination with a building firm with whom we were more at home.

The Build...

The date was February 5th 1996 and the final part of our house build adventure had begun. The builders had arrived on site and in grey February weather, with even a scattering of snow still on the ground, setting out, that is the positioning and staking out of the plan onto the plot had begun.

Initially, as is normally the case with a timber frame build, things moved amazingly quickly. The foundation trenches were dug and filled with concrete, the blockwork of the strip foundations was built up with the floor joists above the damproof membrane, and then underfloor insulation placed in the joist spaces. By this time we could clearly see the outline of the ground floor and hence the positioning of the house within the plot.

The next stage was probably the most exciting and dramatic part of the build. By the middle of February the first part of the timber frame for the ground floor had been delivered. The frame comes in large pre-completed sections with the outer blue damp proof membrane tacked on. The frame really goes up very quickly. By the beginning of March the first floor frame was going up. By March 5th the roof trusses were fixed, and by the 14th March the whole of the roof was felted. Then, by the 22nd all the windows were in position. So, by this time there was this large blue house shaped 'building' where seven weeks earlier there had been an empty plot and empty space!

Inside the blue house things were also happening but in a more confusing way. As the external frame went up so did the inside framing for the partitions which would become the internal walls of the house. The first floor gallery was in position as a solid walkway and marker in the early structure. Below that the main living area and the kitchen and dining area were clearly identified.

Beyond that there was rather less clarity. There were just so many spindly frames close together that it required considerable effort to work out what was what. Then, the pipes, wires and tubes of various colours started appearing. There were bundles of first fix electricity wires, underfloor heating tubes from the first floor hanging down, and, here and there, various bits of plumbing. I found it somewhat disturbing. Would all the bits really end up in their correct places? Fortunately, Pete had a better appreciation than I did of how things should be, and was entirely confident of it all coming together.

The interior began a rapid transformation from the middle of April as drylining of the interior walls with plasterboard began. Light and order emerged amazingly rapidly. Solid walls which were white and bright lightened up the interior spaces and rooms emerged out of the previous confusion. Now the interior, as well as the exterior, began to seem like a real house.

Meanwhile, outside, the blue house was turning into a red bricked one. Although in a timber framed house the timber frame provides the structural integrity and bears the load of the roof, an outer 'skin' provides weather protection and aesthetic appeal. Usually in this country this outer layer is of brick.

Although the interior of our house is unconventional, in many ways we wanted, and the planning authorities required, that it should fit appropriately into the street. Our Cheshire red brick complements that of the Victorian cottages next door. We also have courses of dentil work (a layer of brick work in which alternative bricks protrude a little from the surface) which is traditional in many older Cheshire houses at mid height and underneath the roofline. Bricking up started in the early part of April and was completed by May 10th. So, from the outside at least, the building now looked like a proper house, although, of course it still had a coat of scaffolding.

Meanwhile, inside, during the latter part of May, came the casting of the base of the hearth. on which the chimney grew quickly from large, white, pre-constructed sections made from concrete and volcanic ash. This chimney structure emerged through the upstairs bathroom and then into the loft. The front of the hearth and chimney breast then acquired a facing of brick. Also a brick chimney appeared through the roof. Not long afterwards, our woodburning stove was delivered and placed in position.

Inside, though, we still didn't have those necessities of a finished house – that is a kitchen and stairs. Access upstairs was by ladder leaned against the gallery. For what seemed like quite a long time I hadn't ventured up there, but as the chimney gained height I decided it was time to investigate this part of the house. The problem of moving from the ladder onto the gallery required, for me, a considerable degree of careful manoeuvring. I wasn't intending to make a habit of this way of going upstairs! But it was worth it this once to get the different view from upstairs, providing a different perspective on the inside of the house, but also a more extensive view outside, over the fields, than I had expected.

The kitchen was installed in the first part of June. I had put quite a bit of effort into the design. I wanted it to work well as a kitchen, be reasonably disabled friendly, and also look good as it would be visible from other parts of the ground floor. A local firm put it together for us to our specification. We chose alder wood cabinets in a shaker style with inset panels to some of the doors in a dark green melamine.

The installation was not wholly without problems. First of all, when it was up we realised that one of the full height pull out cabinets was really in the wrong place functionally and aesthetically. In addition, nobody had noticed that it obscured an electrical socket and a pair of light switches! Fortunately it was moved to another position without too much difficulty.

Then we realised that the counter units were not at the height we had specified. We didn't feel too good asking for a large part of the kitchen be refitted, but it really was necessary. Since they hadn't fulfilled our specification, the installers had to remedy this. In the end, though, the kitchen really lived up to our expectation, another important step on the way to our having a real house.

More essential progress in this direction was having the stairs fitted during the beginning of July. This process also involved some fitting problems. These emerged out of having made some changes to the original plan following some revisions suggested by the fitter – but made on the phone. Making changes by phone is *not* a good idea. In our case the result was newel posts placed in front of two windows near the bottom of the stairs. The intention – improving the balustrade support to make it easier for me to get up the stairs – had been good, but the aesthetic result was disastrous. They had to be removed.

There had been one other earlier adjustment made during the build process, the re-positioning of the Velux window openings above the main living area. Originally placed too high up in the sloping ceiling, we dithered anxiously (at least on my part) about this for some time, then realised that if we didn't act fast we would be stuck with them. The builders were quite ready to make the change, and only charged us an extra £300, small beer in the overall build cost.

Apart from these little 'hiccups' the build itself went pretty well. We had a good ongoing relationship with the builders. By the end of July the build was almost, but not quite there. There were some important things still outstanding, but we didn't see much of the builders through August or into September. We weren't too bothered. We hadn't yet sold our previous house so weren't ready to move. We also had some important things to do at the house, and were quite happy to be there without the builders around.

Our Contribution…

Clearly, the builders had been doing by far the greater part of the work of the actual construction. Yet, it still felt very much our build, and our house in a way that was completely different from our experience with our previous house which we had also bought from new. That had been a standard estate house, and although we had visited it during the final stages of its building we could only have very minimal input.

As described earlier this new self-build house was *ours* because we had designed it to suit our needs and preferences. It was exciting and fulfilling to experience design emerge into reality as the build progressed. There was, of course, a degree of worry and anxiety as to whether the completed house would be up to our hopes and expectations. But by the time the spaces had become rooms and living areas, it was clear to us (and friends who came to view) that this was going to be an interesting house.

Our involvement also came through keeping a close track of the build as it progressed. We visited frequently to check progress. Inevitably, there were some bad days, especially at the mid way stage. The house wasn't fully weather proof as quickly as I had expected. The living area floor would be wet and mucky, with used tea bags and cigarette ends scattered around. Would it ever be clean and tidy and finished?

The other involvement was a financial one. We had to ensure that the money came in to pay to the builders at the various agreed build stages. We had a stage mortgage in which the building society released money when the building inspectors had checked on progress. This mostly worked pretty well, although there was one point when things went a little adrift. Somewhat frantic phone calls had to be made to find out what was (or was not) going on – and get the process back on track.

We also had to keep control of the build process in the sense of not allowing too many extras to be incorporated into the build above the original agreed contract price. Pete instituted an 'Extra Over Form' which described any required addition. We and the builders had to sign this before anything could happen. One of the greatest risks in a self-build project is going over budget and it can happen very easily. We were fortunate that no unforeseen problems (such as a requirement for extra foundation work) arose during the build. We were strict with ourselves about not upping the specification as we went along. We knew that with the increased uncertainty introduced by my MS diagnosis it was more important than ever that we kept to budget – and we did so pretty closely.

None of this was actual 'hands-on' contribution, but we had planned we would do something that involved an actual physical contribution to the project. This took the form of the painting and decorating – painting the internal walls and staining the woodwork ourselves, and we started at the beginning of May.

Only gradually did we realised that we had taken on a substantial job. It was easier in some ways than doing redecoration as there wasn't any existing furniture in the way. However, there are quite a lot of walls and plenty of ceilings in a four bedroomed house! We kept at it – working in the evenings and weekends.

All the walls would be the same colour – creamy buttermilk, partly a practical choice. We wouldn't have been able to keep up with the supply chain needed for a complex scheme. The objective was to get the job finished! But it is also an easy to live with, soothing colour, and its use throughout helps to accentuate the inter-connectedness of the parts of the house.

We had also taken on the staining of all the skirting board, door architraves and the stairs – a fiddly job. I couldn't make quite as much of a contribution as I would have done in pre MS days. I sat down as much as I could on the job and had regular rests, but even so I painted the lower two thirds of the walls of most of the house. Pete did the upper third and all the ceilings. I also did a lot of staining, including the whole of the staircase and gallery railings.

Alongside this, Pete was also working very hard at floor level. Instead of carpeting the whole of the house we decided to lay wood effect laminate flooring in a number of the rooms – or rather, Pete would lay it. In the end he did the kitchen, dining and study/library areas, and the downstairs bedroom. Upstairs, he did the study and our bedroom, involving us in quite a few repeat journeys to our nearest Ikea, and much extensive laying work on Pete's part.

Altogether, these occupied us well beyond May. Indeed they took up most of the summer. We didn't have a holiday, but well worth it to feel that, even if we weren't building anything, we were making a real contribution to 'finishing off' the house. The builders were only there infrequently so we began to feel that it was properly our territory now.

At the beginning of September we had a celebration – lighting our first fire in the new woodburning stove. Having taken over a couple of director's chairs, we could sit in quite reasonable comfort. We got ourselves a drink – green tea, rather than champagne! We sat and contemplated the continually varying flames, an important moment of success and achievement. The fire lit easily and was burning well – we felt it was an important indicator for the future.

Moving In…

In the middle of September we received an acceptable offer for our old house. But the new house wasn't wasn't fully complete! The input of the builders had become somewhat dilatory over the summer. Vital aspects such as a central heating boiler and some of the plumbing were not yet in place. We had to apply some pressure!

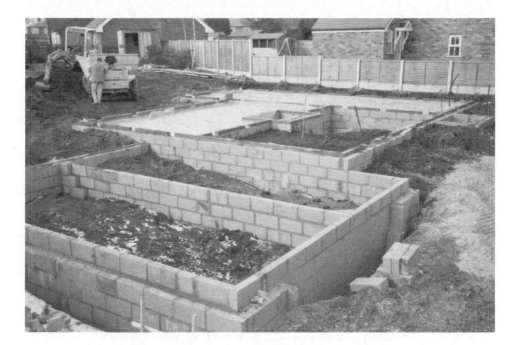

Foundations

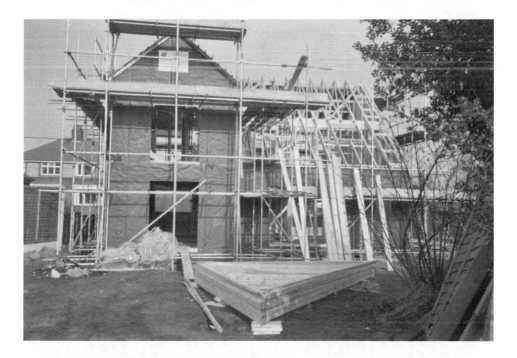

Beginning to be a house

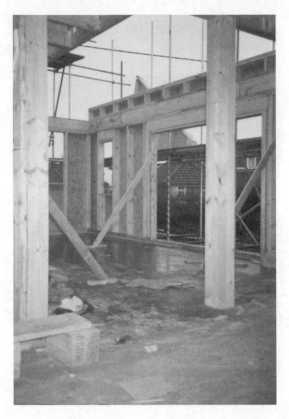

Where's the roof?

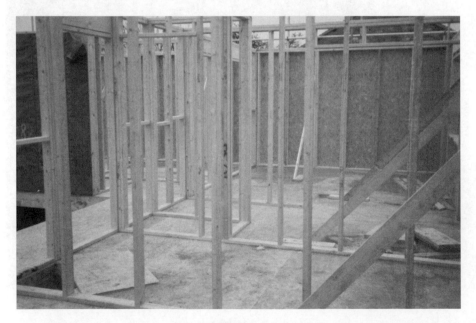

A maze of posts

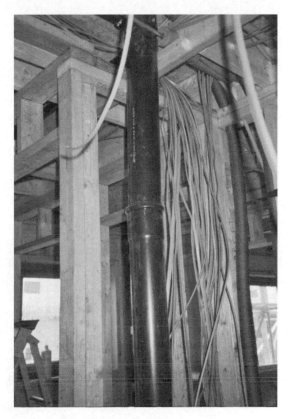

A mess of pipes and cables

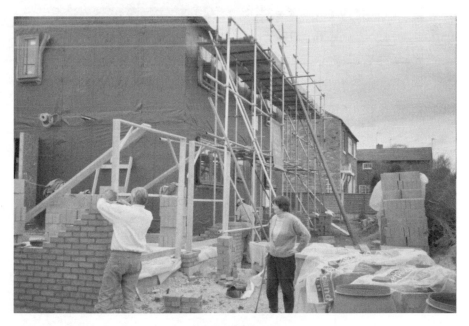

Bricking up

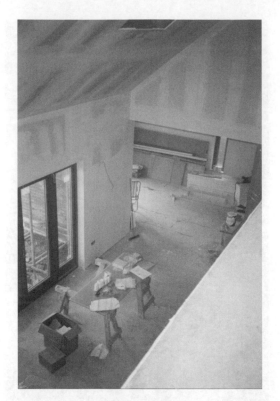

From the gallery

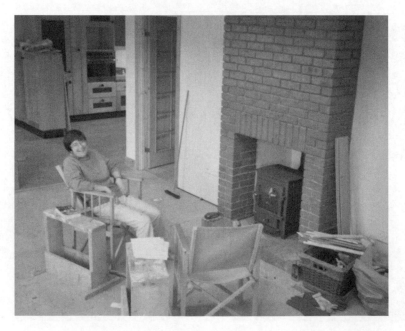

Getting comfortable!

Fortunately, by the time the day for the move came, on November 6th 1996, everything was ready. The move itself went as well as these things can, and we settled in very quickly. Of course, we were moving into an already familiar house. We had previously planned where all the furniture was going to go, indeed, some things had been designed to fit around it such as the floor electric sockets in the living area.

We didn't need a great deal of new furniture, other than a newly bought three seater settee already in position. The covers were multi-coloured – navy blue, shades of olive-green, a dark terracotta red, and some beige and lighter blue, the pattern a kind of zig-zag stripes, but soft and irregular and not hard-edged. Shortly after we bought a large commodious coffee table, stained in olive, to go in front.

Since then we have replaced our old, brown, two-seater with a second three-seater sofa in dark red. The pair of sofas are placed at right angles to the stove, and to the French windows. On winter evenings the focus is towards the ever-changing flames. In the summer it is out towards the garden.

When we moved in we did make one change from our original intentions, that our four bedrooms would enable us to have a study each. However, during the build we had realised that the upstairs room with French windows and a token balcony rail, looking over the garden, was going to provide such a pleasant space that it would be difficult to decide who should have it. Fortunately, as a good sized room we solved the problem by agreeing to share it.

Moving in and getting settled was hugely satisfying. The house did, and still does, live up to our hopes and dreams. There aren't many benefits to contracting MS but one has been getting a more exciting, innovative and enjoyable house than would otherwise have been the case.

Although the original objective of the ground floor open-plan arrangement was to accommodate possible wheel chair use, we just enjoy it and find it a very pleasant and sociable arrangement, not only for us two, but also when we have friends around. We've found that unusually, there are views and vistas within the house. From the living area we can see through to the dining area, part of the kitchen, and the library area; from the kitchen there is a view through to the back garden; from upstairs on the gallery one can overlook a goodly part of the ground floor. The elevated ceiling over the living area makes for a very roomy and open feeling all around, and the French windows, together with the veluxes make for a very light house.

One of the most important things to do as part of the moving in process was to get our grandfather clock positioned and set up. The clock is a very precious possession, inherited from Pete's grandmother who lived in Manchester. It is a Manchester made clock dating from around the 1740s.

In 1968 Pete and his mother transported the clock down to Devon on the roof rack of an A35 van. It wasn't the most respectful way to treat an ancient clock, and unfortunately there was a small mishap! The updraft from a passing lorry led to the clock door being ripped off its hinges. It was rescued, but not before it had been run over by another lorry.

The full restoration of the clock took place after Pete and I were married, and the clock had been transported back up the motorway to Alsager. This time we made sure that it wasn't put on a roof rack! Instead we somehow squeezed it into our first, rather small, new car – a Citroen 2CV.

Our very good friend Ian, who is also a clock enthusiast and has furniture restoration skills, gave important help with the completion of the project. Ian taught history and american studies at Crewe+Alsager. He was not part of the immediate Independent Studies group but we got to know each other well as a result of working together on a programme for supporting student learning skills.

For the restoration Pete bought a piece of new oak, and cut it to the shape of the old door, which we still possessed. The most difficult job he undertook was removing the mahogany inlay from around the margin of the old door and fitting it onto the new one. A few new pieces were needed to finish off. Ian stained the new door to match the old one and applied a French polish finish. A clock repairer contact of Ian's in Shrewsbury completed the final restoration of the mechanism.

The clock had been functioning for quite a few years in our previous two houses. We think, though, that it has its best and most imposing position in our new home. When you come in through our hallway and through the door into the open plan living area, the clock is straight ahead of you, on the right of the French window. It is shown off to its best effect because of the high cathedral ceiling above it.

Living in the house also enabled us to more fully appreciate the positioning of the house and the views to the outside. We can see further over the countryside from the upstairs to the side and front than I had expected. Also, we see some excellent sunsets to the back of the house in the winter. I have become much more aware of the seasonal movement of the position of the setting sun – sunset views are less good in summer because the setting sun disappears behind neighbouring houses.

Having said that, neighbouring houses intrude amazingly little into views from the house. From the living area our view into the garden involves a side view of the dormer bungalow which adjoins a part of the end of our garden. Beyond that we can see part of a second bungalow, but the rest of the houses on that side of the street are out of sight. The bungalows on the other side of the road are completely out of sight behind our side hedge. Over the hedge at the end of the garden we can see to a group of mature trees beyond the end of the road.

So, we have been hugely lucky. The plot I discovered was really quite an exceptional one and the house we have built on it suits us exactly.

Things Outside…

So, our new home was complete, and occupied, and being enjoyed. But as with all new houses, the outside surroundings, what would become a garden, were in a rather different condition. Fortunately we had had much of the area in front of the house and garage paved as part of the build process, so we weren't traipsing dust or mud into the house. But otherwise, the ground had that 'leftover from building' look.

At the front of the house, on either side of the drive area, there were two large depressions which would need filling in. At the back we had decided that we wanted to have a pond so quite early on Pete began to dig this out. Unlike the garden makeover programmes, this was not a fast job. Pete just kept at it whenever he had a little bit of spare time and it wasn't raining. He barrowed the spoil out to the front. Very gradually the hole in the back garden got bigger and those in the front were filled in.

Meanwhile we had persuaded the builders to come back to do a further job for us. This was to construct a deck adjacent to the back of the house. It was instead of, but better than, having a patio. The advantage for me was that I would be able to walk straight out through the French windows, rather than having to negotiate steps – which I would find difficult without the provision of a handrail. Having the deck meant that there was somewhere to sit outside – even if there wasn't yet too much of a beautiful view.

By the summer of 1998 we had a deck and a pond with water in it! Pete and Ian had together fitted a liner into the big hole, laid some stones, rocks even, to make one side of the pond at an angle to the deck. The excavation for the pond goes a little way under the deck, so, with the liner fitted and the pond filled, the water extends underneath. On the third side of the pond a pebble beach was constructed to allow birds to come down to drink and bathe. Finally, a board walk extension to the deck passes above the pebbly beach, turns the corner and provides an apparent bridge to form the fourth side of the pond. The ideas for the structure and arrangement of the pond evolved, rather than being planned from the start. We are rather pleased with the way it has turned out.

The remaining part of the garden, beyond the pond, was constructed in the summer of 2000. Conveniently a small endowment policy matured in time to provide the funds, so we had landscape contractors to do this work. The bridging boardwalk from the pond now continues as a curving, flagged path which extends to the far corner of the garden where it expands to provide a small sitting area with a different view over the garden. An area of shingle planting and a raised bed fill in the space between the pond and the new sitting area. The completed garden feels quite splendid – although now we have a new problem since it is beginning to become somewhat over-grown!

An Energy Efficient House?

As indicated at the beginning of this chapter, one of our aims in pursuing the self-build approach was to have an energy efficient house with heating bills as low as possible. We did have some thoughts about going further. The highest aim identified by the real enthusiasts is building an autonomous house – one independent of external services. This requires electricity generation (solar or wind), water collection from the roof, grey water recycling and composting toilets, as well as an energy efficient structure.

We did make some investigation into composting toilets, but these were rejected because of the need to have a basement, which would have pushed up the building costs considerably. We got a little further with grey water recycling, and the necessary pipes are largely in place. It was my, probably over-anxious, concerns about foaming loo flushes which stopped us going the whole way with this! Ultimately, our green objectives were more conventional, resting in our attempts to have a house that is as energy efficient as possible.

There were four components to our attempt to achieve this. The first one of these had nothing to do with anything we or the builders did – it was a consequence of the siting and positioning of the house. The rear of the house faces towards the south west, and so the French windows to the living area lead to a moderate amount of solar gain on sunny winter days. The second and most obvious strategy was to ensure that we had high levels of insulation in the walls, floor and roof. We also have a mechanical ventilation system with heat recovery because quite a bit of heat can be lost through window ventilators and, of course, double glazing. Our heating uses a gas condensing boiler seen as the most efficient system. Under floor central heating also makes a contribution in two ways. The complex electronic controls give us six different heating zones. Also, the gentle heat from the whole of the floor avoids hot and cold spots and allows as to run the heating at a lower temperature than for a conventional radiator system.

So does the system actually work more efficiently? It is quite difficult to prove this because we do not have a controlled comparison. However, there is some suggestive evidence and experience. When we compared gas consumption for the previous smaller house and our new dwelling, we found that we were using less gas in the new one.

Other information came from major problems we experienced with our first condensing boiler. This gave us a lot of trouble with lengthy breakdowns, being out of action for around six week periods during the winters of 2000 and 2001. So with no central heating the problem was how to achieve replacement warmth.

The wood burning stove provided our salvation! We had bought this only to provide the pleasures of real flames in the evening. Indeed we had chosen the smallest model because we thought that otherwise, with our efficient insulation and the central heating having been on during the day, it might be too warm.

With the central heating out of action we kept the stove burning all day, and all night – after stoking it up last thing before we went to bed. Kept in like this, it gives out a lot of heat. As recommended for energy efficient homes our chimney goes up through the centre of the house. The whole of the brick chimney breast would be hot, and upstairs where the covered in chimney goes through the main bathroom, the wall around it would be warm. The whole downstairs living area stayed at a good comfortable temperature – our open plan arrangement had another benefit! Even upstairs it was quite acceptably warm and we didn't need to use supplementary heating.

Of course, it was quite hard work because the wood supply had to be kept up continuously and the fire fed. We have two log baskets so one is always full. Fortunately, in both years we had good supplies of wood which we keep stacked up behind the garage. In many ways it was really quite pleasant having the stove going all day in miserable winter weather – but then I wasn't the one who had to do the chopping and supplying!

Since 2001 we have taken a different kind of step forward in relation to energy autonomy. We are now generating some of our own electricity. In the spring of 2004 we used a bequest from Pete's uncle to finance the installation of 16 photo voltaic panels on our roof.

Of course one of the problems with such panels is that they are not necessarily generating the electricity at the time that you most need it. Our panels are connected in to the national grid system. One of the electricity companies buys our electricity when we have a surplus, and we get electricity from them in the usual way when we are not generating anything. The expectation is that over the course of the year we should generate about as much as we consume, even if we can't always use it directly.

In 2004 we felt that we were doing a little bit of important pioneering. The urgent need to counteract global warming means that alternative approaches to electricity generation are required. Increased use of photo voltaic technology has the potential to make some contribution.

Chapter Six

Exercise is Good Medicine

Staying Active…

From the start of getting MS I was determined to stay as active as I possibly could. Exercise is important for anybody but I felt that it was particularly so for me, partly because I was used to taking and enjoying exercise. I didn't want to lose that if I could help it. Secondly, I knew that if I didn't take much exercise I would rapidly lose fitness and muscle tone. Then if things did improve in terms of my MS it might be difficult to fully realise and take advantage of that improvement. One particular statement from Judy Grayham's self help guide to coping with MS epitomises that judgement. This reads 'Regular exercise can make the difference between being able to stand and walk – or becoming wheelchair bound'.

The initial period when I had to adapt to physical incapacity was immediately after the initial relapse in the summer of 1993. Looking back, that period of restriction was over relatively quickly. Nevertheless, the exercise approaches I adopted and developed during that time have proved their worth in my later coping.

My first strategy, as soon as I started the subsequent period of sick leave, was to make sure that I had a short daily walk around the estate where we lived. Initially, of course, I couldn't walk very well or very far. I needed to use my stick for support, and to ensure that I was secure against a sudden loss of balance, at any time. However, I soon tried to walk a few steps holding the stick off the ground. Then I tried to extend this so that I was just using the stick as I got tired, or when I came to a kerb or any other kind of unevenness. However, by October 14th, around two and a half months after it had all started, I recorded that I took my stick on my daily walk, but didn't use it at all. I felt that this was an important achievement and, most especially, an indicator that things really were improving.

Of course, I was walking far more slowly than I would have done previously and that was frustrating. I didn't walk very far either – my usual walk through October and into November was about half a mile. Then I began to gradually extend the distances. I had to be careful not to exhaust myself before I got home, but I began to seek out places where I could sit and have a rest – usually on somebody's garden wall. So, as we got through November I was walking a mile and slightly more.

Another area of physical activity where I had already made progress was in swimming. Having previously been quite a good swimmer I hadn't felt there was any great risk attached to this – although I felt newly vulnerable to those kinds of swimmers who thrash up and down the baths without taking a great deal of care over who they might meet on the way. I was pleased to find that there were special recuperative swimming sessions provided at the local baths. These were intended for people suffering some degree of physical infirmity, or convalescing after illness. So I joined a group of enthusiastic but civilised swimmers who took care not to meet too abruptly in the middle of the pool. I am surprised, checking back, that as early as October 11th in 1993 I noted in my diary that I had done 18 lengths.

A new activity which we took up at this time was Yoga. Pete came with me to evening sessions at the local comprehensive. I had, in the past, thought that the practice of yoga would be worth trying, but had never quite got round to it. Now I had read that yoga had positive benefit in relation to MS. It is a gentle, rather than aggressive form of exercise. But it does involve some positions which require a certain degree of balancing, and balance is a problem for many people with MS.

I did feel a little uncertain and vulnerable to begin with. However, one of the advantages of yoga is that it is not competitive in any way. I could position myself next to a wall so that there was support available as necessary. If a position was clearly going to be impossible for me, I could just sit it out. As with the other forms of exercise I was taking, things did improve. We started to do half an hour's yoga most evenings before our evening meal, something that I have kept up reasonably regularly since.

So things did improve quite quickly. I was lucky that there were activities that I could go back to and get involved in. The number of lengths swum and the distance walked provided clear indicators of progress. These markers showing real improvement were hugely encouraging. Although I still didn't feel that I could walk easily or comfortably at least it did seem that some improvement was taking place.

It might appear from some of these comments that progress in regaining mobility was checked off and measured in a primarily objective way, but it was also a matter of pleasure and enjoyment – of taking great satisfaction in doing again those things I had once taken for granted, and for a while, feared I might never be able to do again.

I walked other places besides around the block – mostly at the weekend with Pete. We discovered or rediscovered some local possibilities that formerly would have been dismissed as being rather flat and boring. We enjoyed gentle ambles along a nearby canal. We got to know a couple of local country parks, one of which was well wooded and very spectacular on a sunny autumn day. And it wasn't really flat at all. There was a small lake with views towards the Peak District hills and a substantial stream with waterfalls and quite precipitous banks in places but, most importantly, a good, accessible path.

So, by the time December came my ability to get around was a great deal improved. It was by no means back to normal, but I could walk much more easily and for increasing distances. Over the remainder of 1994 we tried to keep up the walking as much as we could. I think that over this period, and into 1995 we were in many ways more active than we had been in pre-MS days, although a somewhat different pattern of activity. In terms of walking in particular, we would previously have had a day out in the Peak District once every three or four weeks, when we would have done a walk of around eight, ten or eleven miles. Now, we usually walked locally – along the canal, or at one of the nearby country parks, but we did this a lot more often than we had taken our longer walks previously. If the weather was at all reasonable we would try to get out most weekends – we felt we had to make the most of this walking ability.

We did so – not only in our local area but also in the holidays we took during this period. As I've mentioned, we had a wonderfully enjoyable holiday in Switzerland in the late Spring of 1994, and a real walking holiday in the Lake District in Easter 1995.

Curtailment...

But, as I've also reported, this was only a short term return to my pre MS level of activity. From the Autumn of 1995 and onwards there was a slow and insidious decline in my ability to walk. I was soon back to using a stick most of the time. After quite short distances my left leg seemed to lose appreciation of how it was meant to act in this walking business. I had always to be thinking about where I could take a rest. Since there aren't always convenient rest stations available, we took to carrying a folding stool with us.

Determined to keep going, I didn't stop going for walks altogether, but by the middle of 1996 I was down to about a quarter of a mile – and then I required a rest. The other feature of my walking at that time was that I was doing it more and more slowly. My diary records the frustration I was feeling. There was just nothing I could do to speed up. It was completely beyond my power to move any faster.

I was still able to keep swimming, but was very conscious that I was doing it less well. I had particular difficulty doing the leg movement of breast stroke. I could keep up the leg movement of crawl since it is a very simple up and down kick. But crawl is a more energetic stroke so even though I tried to take it easy it made me very tired. Then I would have some difficulty in hauling myself out of the pool at the end of my swim. After that there was the business of getting dressed again! I have never seen this as a favourite part of the process of going swimming. It is worse when you have to take the greatest of care not to slip as you move around, and actions feel clumsy and convoluted.

By this time I was either having to drive into the university, or get a lift from Pete or somebody else. Although the swimming pool was only across the road from my work place, I was increasingly unable to walk back after my swim. At the same time it just reinforced feelings of incapability to have to take the car that short distance. Anyway, I didn't always have the car. We only had the one and sometimes Pete needed it. There wasn't any particular crisis which stopped me from swimming, and I kept it up through most of 1996. However, I wasn't getting quite the same level of enjoyment as previously and my enthusiasm and motivation dwindled away – as did my commitment.

So, keeping active and maintaining the exercise was clearly becoming more difficult. Fortunately, during this difficult period, there was the ongoing distraction of our new house, which was gradually taking shape. Alongside this I was still walking and doing yoga, but clearly some re-assessment was becoming necessary if I was to maintain mobility.

Adjustments Required...

So what could be done? There were clearly limitations. To some extent I just had to be more patient – get used to going slowly – take positive pleasure in the fact that I could still walk, though it was easier to do this out in the country at the weekend, rather than battling to get around the university during the week.

The other strategy was to experiment more with walking aids. I bought myself a pair of yellow crutches with the hope that they might enable me to walk a little faster. I practised with them at weekends. I did use them for a while but in the end they were discarded and have stayed in the walking stick container for a long time now. They seemed clumsy to use, made holding things more difficult and didn't really help with speeding up to any substantial degree. Impatience and exasperation ruled!

What I did, in the end, find much more useful was a stick with a Fischer handle. These have handles which are shaped to receive the palm of your hand – they come in left and right handed versions. With a good, sturdy ferrule I found this much more secure than the stick I had used previously – there was a good solid base on which to lean.

But one has to be careful not to lean too much and get out of balance. It took me a while to be convinced that I needed two sticks – couldn't I walk quite well with just the one? It was my mother's suggestion that I try a second, and I resisted it for a while. But she was right. You are more secure with two, especially on rough ground, and I think it *is* possible to walk a little faster. You are also better balanced with two sticks. With just one it is easy to find yourself, without at all meaning to, leaning too much on that one. With the two you can more easily take up a better balanced position and a more natural gait. I don't use the two sticks all the time – only when I am going for a proper walk, but I have no doubt of their value in those circumstances. And they are invaluable in those fortunately rare occasions when a large dog decides to be over-friendly!

I could, and did, still walk – but it was a frustrating business. I wanted to get out and not feel totally exhausted after a short distance. I especially wanted to be able to get out to beautiful places and not just be viewing them from a seat in a car. So, the time came, in the summer of 1996, when I began to feel that I would need to acquire a wheelchair.

Not an easy decision to make – it involved personal admission that the MS was seriously restricting my mobility. It also required an acceptance that there was no sign of it getting better, and that the limitations were likely to be here to stay. At the same time there were positive aspects. I was going to be using the wheelchair on my own terms. It would enable me to go to places and do things that wouldn't otherwise be possible. I certainly wouldn't (at least for the present) be giving up walking. I would be a part-time wheelchair user.

So, I became a wheelchair owner. It was a lightweight, folding model, but one I hoped would be reasonably strong and resistant to the rough treatment I expected to give it. It was probably the brochure picture of an attractive young lady wheeling down a wooded lane and the name 'Actif' which sold me this particular model! My choice of a chair on which the enamelled parts were in bright yellow was also intended as some sort of statement.

I was pleased with my acquisition. It did, as I had hoped, improve my countryside mobility – at least to a degree. It enabled us to get back to visiting local countryside parks, where paths were generally quite well surfaced. I soon adopted a strategy of walking a bit while pushing the chair, and then riding when I got tired. I didn't really like to be pushed – not even by Pete. But, of course, there were times when this was the best policy. Wheeling by pushing the wheel hand rims is hard work.

Despite some mixed feelings, the wheelchair had been a good

purchase. But it still wasn't allowing me to get into the countryside to the extent that I wished. Unless you get into serious training there is a limit to how far you can go – and it's hard work for the pusher too, especially if you want to go uphill. It is also difficult, pretty well impossible really, to use a conventional wheelchair over rough or uneven ground.

So, were there any other possibilities? While researching the wheelchair options I had come across a commentary on the use of electric battery powered scooters or buggies as a means of more serious cross country transport. The writer commented on using his buggy to explore both the Hebridean Islands and the Black Forest in Germany doing 20 mile off road 'rambles'. This sounded more like what I was after. Some further research into available models led to the purchase, later in August 1997, of a Lark 6 buggy which could supposedly manage 8 mph.

Initially, I used the buggy a fair bit. We had some good rides on Forestry Commission routes in particular, which are now being opened up for recreational use. They have the advantage over the usual countryside paths of being well surfaced, and not degenerating into narrow trails which would now be impassable. The other major advantage is they don't have stiles. Getting over the stiles used to be just an accepted part of a country walk. Using a buggy means that they are totally impossible – one just has to turn back. Forestry Commission trails mean that free buggy passage is pretty well guaranteed.

Forestry routes sometimes have the disadvantage that they can be dark passageways through the uniform, serried ranks of towering conifers. However, there are better possibilities – and inspiring views to be had. One of our best expeditions with the buggy came on a sunny October weekend visit to Llandudno in 1997.

We drove up the Conwy valley and took one of the single track roads into the Gwydyr forestry area. There are some splendid views from the road as one can see the mountains of Snowdonia on the skyline to the west. We parked just above a small reed-fringed boggy pool.

We set off with me riding the buggy and Pete walking. Our objective was another larger lake probably not much more than a mile distant as the crow flies but a fair bit further on the winding forestry tracks. Route finding is not that easy since there is no way marking or sign posting and it is not always easy to get correspondence between the tracks and the ordnance survey map. But it was a beautiful day, and we weren't in a hurry. We got to the lake in time for a picnic lunch down on its pebbly beach, and enjoyed its quiet, isolated situation and the view along its length. The lake (Llyn y Parc) cannot be reached by road and so getting there felt like a considerable achievement.

Llandudno itself is quite good for wheelchair wheeling. The main promenade is wide and smooth, somewhere where hand propelled progress is easy and enjoyable. The western promenade is not quite so smooth, but it does have the most splendid views towards the mountains.

Locally, in rides from our house, the buggy also had advantages. I could vary my walking route a little by riding the buggy so far, and then abandoning it and walking further on foot. It also allowed me to get into town without using the car. It meant that I could ride around town to do various bits of shopping, rather than having to park the car and walk, and get tired walking around. I soon realised though that one has to be careful about one's route – 'bumping down' over the kerb is not a good idea.

However, I soon found that the buggy had a few problems and limitations. It wasn't as efficient as I had expected in getting up hills. The supposed 8 mph capability soon declined on an uphill gradient. If the battery was low there was a real risk of the machine failing altogether. It wasn't that reliable. On one occasion, coming home from town the buggy just stopped, and there was nothing I could do to get it moving again. I was stuck! Marooned!

So what to do? I couldn't just sit and wait. Nobody would be able to help because the machine is too heavy too push. The only possibility seemed to be to abandon the vehicle and walk! Fortunately I wasn't that far from home – somewhere in the region of half a mile. I just about managed to get back without collapsing on the pavement. When I had reached home and recovered I actually felt quite pleased with myself because I had walked further than I had for a while. I phoned the local police to inform them about the abandoned buggy but they didn't seem that bothered.

That sort of experience didn't give me a great deal of confidence, so the buggy was completely abandoned when I discovered better alternatives. But, looking back I can more fully appreciate the value of electric buggies to many disabled people. They have become more commonly used since I had mine in 1997. The range of different kinds of models is much wider, and I hope the reliability of the batteries has improved – it certainly shouldn't be beyond the bounds of current technology!

A rather different practice, which I began to take up at this time, was not to do with mobility, and although it required to be practised it did not involve exercise either. This was meditation. I bought an introductory guide to meditation and decided to have a try. I used the approach of meditating 'on the breath' which we had tried a little at the end of our yoga classes. For me, as I think for many others, the experience of 'pulling back' attention and concentration to the breath, after it has become diverted, is as important as the experience of concentration and focus itself.

I haven't kept up my practice of meditation quite as effectively as my practice of actual exercise. There have been periods when it has lapsed completely. Nevertheless I have come back to it. It is difficult to identify clear beneficial outcomes, but it does give me a sense of satisfaction and I think that there are subtle but still important benefits.

Taking a Walk…

This discussion of wheelchairs and electric buggies might be giving the impression that I am no longer walking anywhere. I am glad to say that this is not true. My walking ability is still severely limited – a mile is about my absolute maximum in the best of conditions. 1996 to 1997 was the worst period, but I still kept walking a little. This was either with the wheelchair (part walking and pushing, and part riding), as described previously, or very short walks from our house using crutches or sticks. Fortunately, things have improved somewhat since then.

As I have already written, in November 1996 we moved house. Our new home has a whole host of positive qualities. One of these is not to do with the house itself, but with its position. Not much further than just across the road, our road actually becomes a single track lane. The houses are left behind and there are fields on either side. I soon feel that I am really in the country. Having this kind of opportunity so near at hand really helped me to keep walking.

The lane is a popular walk for many neighbours. I often meet other people during the completion of my own walk. There are particular people whom I know I am likely to meet at certain times. We can stop and catch up with news, so my walk is partly a social experience. I don't manage a walk every day, but I do try to get out as much as possible when the weather is at all reasonable.

What is it about the lane itself that appeals to me? A crucial characteristic is that, although a little rough and potholed in places, it does have a hard, bitumised surface. Soft, uneven ground demands much greater walking effort and is more difficult for me to deal with. As a single track road, with a relatively poor surface, which doesn't go anywhere in particular there is also limited traffic. It is usually fairly quiet and peaceful and I can enjoy the lane and the countryside views in a leisurely kind of way.

There are of course some cars, and inevitably some which go much too fast. There are also, at some periods, huge tractors almost filling the whole width of the lane. They have trailers of muck, grass for silage or crushed maize, depending on the season. I need to keep alert and have a plan for getting out of the way fairly smartly. For part of the lane there are reasonable verges so it is easy to get on to these quite quickly. On the narrower parts where the banks and hedges go straight up one has to get in tight and sideways on.

But, to get back to the lane itself – for me this lane is not just any lane. It has, to my mind, the varied qualities of an ideal lane. It is not flat and arrow straight as some lanes in Cheshire are. It meanders gently around a number of curves, so that at no point can you see along it very far. The first section is fairly flat, bounded on either side by hawthorn hedges. But then there are two gates on either side. On one side there is a view downhill and across the fields. On the other you can see to the very beginning of the Peak District hills.

The lane then begins to slope gradually downhill where the road bridges a small stream. For quite a long time this was as far as I could manage and I would sit and rest on the stonework of the bridge. Now, I can climb back up the bank on the other side and then around the gentle curve to the T junction. There is a huge beech tree just to the side and, since this is something of a high spot, views around. On summer evenings, if I get there at the appropriate time, and weather conditions are right, I often have a splendid view of the sunset. At other times, and on any part of the walk, I can enjoy the varied cloudscapes. These days I notice and appreciate the skies more than I used to.

Up to this point I will usually feel I have been walking pretty well. I might think I've been walking quite fast. I won't have been leaning too much on the sticks – just trying to touch them lightly to the ground. On the return journey this gradually gets more difficult and I find myself leaning more heavily – even if I'm consciously trying not to. Gradually too my speed and pace fall off. I have to be on guard against my left leg dragging. The smoothness of my walking declines and is more out of control. My left leg especially gets tired and heavy so that, on some days, it can be difficult to force one foot in front of the other.

Other days are better – or the sun is shining and I just feel like going further. Then I can decide to go beyond the T-junction. In one direction I then pass an attractive old farmhouse with cobbled yard and interesting looking but somewhat tumble-down barns. The house is a grade II listed building with partly Tudor origins which has recently been sympathetically restored. Beyond is an overgrown pond – it has really pretty well disappeared in the time I've been walking here. Then there is a set of four attractive Victorian terraced cottages – hardly long enough to be called a row, really. Beyond, you get back to the main road. I do, on occasion get this far. It is just over half a mile. The lane continues across the main road, but I know that if I attempted to go further I would not be able to get back home.

The other arm of the 'T' leads down an avenue of mature, well-grown trees. The horse chestnuts are particularly attractive and in the early autumn I enjoy searching for conkers in among the leaves. Unfortunately the trees are gradually being lost – two have come down in storms since we moved here. This arm provides the drive to Tall Chimneys – a large, rambling Victorian vicarage that does indeed have tall and dramatic chimneys. From the final part of the public right of way there are extensive, sweeping views. On a very good day it is possible to see over to the Bickerton hills, almost across the other side of the Cheshire plain. The right of way path turns off the drive to cross fields behind Tall Chimneys and down into the valley beyond. Here there is an attractive, but often very muddy riverside walk. I have been there, but even with present improvements I cannot do so on my own.

If I have had an extended walk down one of the arms of the T, then I will be pretty tired, even exhausted, when I get home and be fit for nothing until I have had a rest. Sometimes, I feel thoroughly exasperated at being so exhausted after having walked such a short distance. I bemoan the fact that without my MS I would be able to extend my walk into a number of longer and attractive routes. But mostly, I celebrate the pleasure of the walk, feel pleased that I am able to take a walk when I choose to, and when the weather is right. I think about how hugely lucky I am to have such a splendid lane to walk down immediately at my front door.

Moving to the Music…

In June 1997 we went to a friend's 50th birthday party. Since this was the celebration of an old school friend of mine, and away from our home base, we didn't actually know that many people – but it was a very friendly and enjoyable occasion. Then the music began. A local folk band was playing and calling the directions. I would have loved to have been able to join in. It was hard to sit on the sidelines – but risking taking a fall in such a situation was not sensible.

After the band had finished we had pop music from the sixties and seventies instead. Since in this situation one can dance vigorously – or very gently and sedately – I began to think that maybe I could join in and have a go.

The feeling of wanting to try was very strong. I persuaded Pete that if we held hands to help my balance, and did some very gentle moving around to the music, then it was probably safe. It was, and with good rests in between we had a few 'dances'. I was really pleased. It was not that I had particularly missed dancing. In our middle age there hadn't been that many opportunities for taking part, and certainly since the start of my MS there hadn't previously been the sort of occasion when I felt I had the opportunity. Now there had been, and even if rather tentatively, I'd had a go!

But, how often would there be other such opportunities? There wouldn't be many unless I did something to organise them for myself.

I decided to have a go at putting on appropriate CDs at home. Initially I was rather tentative about it. It did mean dancing without a supporting handhold from Pete. I didn't feel that secure, and I was quite careful and restrained in the movements I made. However, very gradually my dancing capabilities improved. As 1998 moved into 1999, I could feel myself becoming more confident about the movements I was making, and more ready to test out my balance. I haven't fallen at all while I've been 'moving to the music'. It has been one indicator that my ability to move around has improved at least a little.

Now, in 2008, I 'have a hop' probably two or three times a week – around 10 minutes, or two or three tracks at a time. I have a stack of CDs on the player so that I can vary the music easily – it is mostly music from the sixties and seventies. Lone dancing might seem a bit of an odd thing to do, but I enjoy it as a small contribution to the variety of my day. As you listen to the lyrics and move around to the beat it is difficult to be sad and miserable.

So, these private 'hops' have a number of advantages and benefits. They can help maintain or increase positive mood. They provide convenient home based exercise whatever the weather. Even short dancing 'spots' can get the heart rate up and so provide some degree of cardiac work-out. And dancing is weight bearing exercise with benefits in relation to osteoporosis prevention.

The other possible benefit is that of helping to improve my balance. Practice is one way of improving balance for anyone. The balance problems experienced by many people with MS are more exteme but there are expert suggestions that practice can be beneficial here too. I'm not sure that dancing to pop music would be on conventional lists of ways of improving balance, but I certainly feel that it helps me. Overall then, I think that having one's own private dance is an enjoyable, and easily controllable way of getting some useful exercise. Although it is unlikely to suit everybody, I think that it could well benefit people with chronic illnesses and disabilities other than MS.

Exercise, the Brain and Well-Being...

When we think about the benefits of exercise we are usually considering direct physical benefits. However, exercise, or lack of exercise, also impact upon the brain. This is a fundamental assumption in physiotherapy. The intention is to exercise and rehabilitate the body, but just as important is to rehabilitate the brain after injury or disuse.

Although there are many remaining limitations and mysteries, our understanding of brain processes and functioning has developed rapidly over recent years. This increased understanding has been supported by better ways of investigating what is going on in the working brain.

I am not the kind of psychologist who has a particular expertise in this area. However, I have been fascinated to read about some of these developments in a very interesting book written for the general reader. This is *Mind Sculpture* by Ian Robertson,[1] who is a psychologist, but also 'one of the world's leading researchers on brain rehabilitation'. Although MS is barely mentioned in the book I would still recommend it as an interesting and encouraging read for anybody who has MS – and for anybody else for that matter.

It is clearly quite impossible to give any kind of overview of the book in the space available, but a couple of points and examples related to use/disuse and damage could be of interest. The first example relates to what happens to the brain when an ankle joint is immobilised through injury. It was found that the area of brain tissue that is devoted to the function of moving this joint actually decreases, and the more so when the ankle is in plaster. These changes would be reversed on recovery, and in the research were reversed earlier by asking patients to practice tensing of the relevant muscles.

Another investigation along similar lines involved anaesthetising some of the fingers of one hand. Prior to this the 'brain map' for the control of the whole hand had been plotted. After anaesthetisation the brain control areas were re-plotted. It was found that the brain areas controlling the non anaesthetised fingers expanded into the control areas for the anaesthetised fingers.

It seems that 'use it or loose it' operates at brain level, as well as in terms of muscle tone and joint flexibility. Long term disuse would seem likely to exacerbate any damage already caused by the MS. These investigations, and many others described by Ian Robertson, certainly reinforced my motivation to keep moving and keep active as far as that is possible.

Why is exercise so important to me? There are quite a number of reasons. Firstly, there is abundant evidence that exercise is good for me (and everybody else). Exercise is likely to contribute substantially to the prevention of cardio-vascular problems – it is good for your heart. There is also some evidence that it has a preventative effect in relation to some cancers and for diabetes.

These preventative effects are of course well known. But it is getting people to actually do the exercise which is the major health education problem. Many people just don't get up and get active. As a disabled person who *is* exercising I can feel pleased that I am giving myself the various health benefits. I can also feel a little superior that I am doing better than all those able bodied people who are not bothering.

To a degree, I perhaps have stronger incentives than the able-bodied to keep exercising. I know that it is particularly important for me, as a disabled person, to maintain muscular strength and tone as far as I can. It is likely that it would be a harder task for me to regain these if they were lost. Also, as a person with MS, in particular, I know that exercise, especially muscle stretching, is likely to be helpful in preventing contractures. Contractures involve the 'freezing' of a joint in a particular position – the normal facility of the joint to bend through its full range of movement is lost. Lack of use is likely to contribute to the development of contractures, but as they develop they will make further movement and exercise more difficult.

Another important feature of the exercise process is that there is increasing evidence that it is linked with psychological as well as physical well-being.[2] There appears to be a positive effect on mood, and links with positive self-esteem. There are also indications that physical activity and exercise are associated with an anti-depressant effect. This linkage is perhaps of particular relevance for people with MS, who are more prone than members of the general population to becoming depressed.

Certainly, for me personally, exercise has important links with enjoyment and positive mood. It gives me a sense of achievement. I feel pleased with myself when I have, say, done my morning exercises or evening yoga. I have feelings of satisfaction and accomplishment in relation to my overall, ongoing exercise participation. It also provides an incentive to get out and about. These outings then give me a great deal of enjoyment as they are happening and pleasure and satisfaction as I look back on them, and talk to others about them.

Perhaps I am now somewhat obsessed with exercise – but I think that it is an obsession worth having. As well as providing pleasure and satisfaction, exercise helps to provide a framework for my day. This framework is certainly not a rigid one but it does give me a set of tasks and targets to aim for. When these are achieved I can feel pleasure and a sense of accomplishment. In many ways I am putting into practice Bandura's ideas about the management of motivation. In psychological terms I am engaging in the self-regulation of my exercise behaviour which allows me to experience self-reinforcement for successful outcomes.

An exercise issue for people with MS relates to the possibility of overdoing it. When I was first diagnosed in 1993 the advice tended to be cautious. One recommendation which I saw was to do less than you know that you can. My attitude has been to do as much as I can manage. Clearly, I do get tired, especially after walking. There will come a point when I need to, indeed have to, stop and take a rest. But I do recover! As far as I can tell, getting tired hasn't done me any harm.

I have been pleased to see that now exercise is much more strongly encouraged in a positive way. Quite a variety of forms of exercise are currently very much encouraged for people with MS – for example horse riding, swimming, canoeing, even climbing.[3] I think that there is also increasing recognition that people with other chronic illnesses can benefit from taking exercise. Of course, common sense, judgement and advice are important, but there is much to be said for 'going for it'.

For myself, as I've said, I have always taken part in various active pursuits. However, in many ways I've become a more dedicated exerciser since becoming ill and disabled. In our skiing days, Pete and I usually had good intentions of doing regular preparatory exercise prior to our skiing trips – but often it didn't happen. Now, I find it easier to sustain the practice – the possibility that maintaining exercise could make a real difference to my continuing mobility is a strong incentive!

Notes and References

1. Robertson, I. (1999). *Mind Sculpture*. London: Bantam Press.
2. For example in the contributions to Biddle, S. J. H., Fox, K. R. & Boutcher, S. H. (Eds) (2000). *Physical Activity and Psychological Well-being*. London: Routledge.
3. See, for example, information on the website of the MS Trust at www.mstrust.org.uk

Chapter Seven

Leaving Paid Employment

It was May 1953 and two men were toiling up the high snow fields of Everest. They had reached the South Summit, 300 feet below the main summit of the mountain. But these were not Hilary and Tenzing. The date was May 26th, not the 29th. The two men were Charles Evans and Tom Bourdillon. They were defeated by faulty oxygen equipment and could not make the final push to the summit to become the first conquerors of Everest.

So, what can the 1953 Everest expedition have to do with my experience? The link is through the post-Everest life of Charles Evans. Formerly a doctor and neurosurgeon, in 1958 he was appointed principal of the then University College of North Wales at Bangor. Very soon afterwards, he was diagnosed with multiple sclerosis. Within five years he was unable to walk, but determined nevertheless to keep working. He retained this demanding and responsible post at Bangor until his retirement in 1984. I found this inspiring and thought that if he could keep working then maybe I could too – in a rather less demanding role.

For the majority of adults, work and employment have a significant place in their lives. It is important at an individual level for a number of reasons. For many it provides a sense of satisfaction and achievement. The work environment is also likely to provide a valuable context for interpersonal contact and the development of friendships. At a more practical level, it enables most of us to make our living.

My job has been an important part of my life. I had worked without any break since I left university. I have also been very fortunate to have had a job which I enjoyed, and found appropriately challenging, but also satisfying. Before the advent of MS, I had every expectation that I would continue to work until retirement age.

To Stay or Not?

After my MS was diagnosed, in 1993, it was very much my intention to keep working – the example of Charles Evans became important. As described earlier, I was able to return to work quite quickly after my initial MS relapse in the summer of 1993. Although there continued to be physical symptoms, and I could never forget that I had MS, it was, in many ways, a case of work as usual.

But then things began to change in a number of ways. Most obviously, as discussed previously, MS began to make its presence clearly felt again. As 1996 progressed, my ability to move around easily and comfortably within the campus became much more constrained.

Outsiders might consider the working life of an academic as a fairly sedentary and static one. In actuality quite a degree of movement from one place to another through buildings and across the campus is required. Of course, I did spend a fair amount of time sitting at my desk – marking essays, preparing lectures, and doing all sorts of administrative tasks. However, equally obviously, I had to be able to move back and forth to a variety of classrooms and lecture theatres some distance away. It is also necessary to get to the library, visit the departmental office, the photocopier, and the offices of other colleagues. Frequently, on these journeys I would need to carry books, files and papers.

In the past, of course, I would take it for granted that I could move from floor to floor within buildings, and from place to place across the campus without any difficulty whatsoever. It would just be a part of the ordinary working day. But as 1996 went on these journeys became more like expeditions for me. I had to work out how I was going to able to carry everything I needed, use my stick, and have a spare hand to get heavy doors open. I needed to take special care that I didn't forget anything at any time, because I wouldn't be able to hurry back to pick it up. Hurrying was no longer an option. I also got tired, and so even slower, quite quickly. Thus, the ordinary business of getting to the right place to do my teaching and other required tasks became much more challenging.

At the same time there were wider changes going on around me which had nothing to do with me personally, but which did have personal implications. These changes involved the organisation of the academic undergraduate degree programmes which were offered in the Crewe+Alsager Faculty. (By this time 'college' had become 'faculty' because Crewe+Alsager, from 1992, had become a constituent part of Manchester Metropolitan University.)

By 1996 the Independent Study Degree had been operating successfully for over fifteen years. During that time we had attracted sufficient students to fill the places we had available, although this became more difficult as the number of places available increased. One problem came from the name of the degree. It was not immediately obvious to students quite what was involved in a degree by independent study. A degree route which involved a named subject or discipline route was a more familiar option. Also we had always attracted a fair proportion of mature students, but with the introduction of fees and loans, times were getting harder for older students and their numbers were decreasing. There were indications that it might become more difficult to maintain full recruitment.

In this context the planned changes in the undergraduate programme had implications for independent study. The Faculty was starting to move to a joint honours degree system. Students would select a pair of degree subjects to be studied jointly over the three degree years. There was thus a fair amount of pressure towards offering Psychology, Sociology, Health Studies etc within this joint honours programme. It was accepted that Independent Study could continue alongside the new system. However, the degree would have difficulty in maintaining its attractiveness alongside the more straightforward subject based options.

As a consequence of the problems arising from my mobility difficulties, and the potential demise of the Independent Study degree, I began to wonder whether I should reconsider my commitment to work. There were two issues, although it was on the first that I focused initially. This was the question of whether I should move from full time teaching to a part-time position.

I spent a few months, from around March 1997, considering the possibility of changing to a part-time post. The obvious advantage would be less work and less pressure, and more non-working time to rest and recuperate. The further question was exactly how much work I should do if I did take a part-time position. I was tending to think in terms of somewhere around a half time post. However, it was more difficult to decide how that work could best be distributed through the week. Typically, a half-time post is concentrated into a two and a half day 'working week'. But another option would be to distribute the lower work load through much of the week – thus working less intensively.

In many ways the latter seemed to have considerable advantage in that it would allow a slower paced working life, with greater time for recovery. However, as I thought about it further I was not so sure. In many ways it could feel more like working as long for half the pay! But, if I decreased the proportion of time I worked much further I would be getting less money than I would on a pension, if I took early retirement.

So, during 1997, I began to contemplate what was the second issue – whether I should give up teaching and take early retirement. This must be one of the most difficult decisions that faces people who become chronically ill, or disabled. There is a whole range of complex pressures and factors involved. It was important to give some attention to working out the pros and cons of the different options.

Various physical problems were emerging at this time. In themselves these did not make working impossible, but they were certainly stressful and made things more difficult. I was beginning to suffer from seriously sluggish bowel action which could delay early morning departure. Some problems with my bladder could also be difficult to manage in the teaching situation. In addition I was suffering periodic intense pain down one side of my body from arm-pit to hip area. Fortunately it didn't last long, but when it was there I think it was the worst pain I had ever felt. When it came, which was a few times over the day, I just had to stop whatever I was doing until it went away again. As previously mentioned I also had an episode of optic neuritis at the end of 1996. This quite seriously affected the sight in my right eye. So, there were times during this period when my body felt that it was 'falling apart', and having been told that I had progressive MS I did wonder what more there was to come. Maybe there was an argument for getting out while I could still enjoy what physical capability remained.

The other pressures were external and part of the changing higher education context. Undoubtedly this was becoming more stressful and the work load was increasing. Staff-student ratios have been going up ever since I started lecturing, but now were putting on a further spurt. So there were more students to be taught, but no more tutors to contribute to the teaching. As a consequence of widened participation rates, students were changing and needed more support in various ways. Teaching and assessment were taking up more time. Alongside this there has been increasing pressure to do research and publish. There were major stresses and strains for everybody, but for me there was the particular concern over the evidence that stress can play a part in the exacerbation of MS.

The above really represented negative reasons for leaving work – they were things to escape from. But when I began to think about it there also seemed to be quite a few opportunities and positive possibilities which would emerge if I did take retirement. Top of my list was the thought it would be much easier to take exercise as and when I wanted to. If the sun was shining I would be able to take advantage and get out and about. Also, I would be able to really enjoy our new home and its surroundings. I could think about doing new and different things, but first of all I would be able to complete the PhD, which I had begun, in a more relaxed way. So, by September 1997 I had made the decision. I was beginning a new stage of my life.

Completing a PhD…

I was fortunate that on leaving employment I was able to get on with an absorbing project which I had already started. I had registered for this PhD during 1995. Clearly, at this stage, I was not embarking on this enterprise for career reasons. It was rather that the opportunity had opened up to achieve a PhD in a way that would allow me to make use of the research I had already been doing for a few years.

The particular opportunity was that Manchester Metropolitan University had recently instituted a scheme whereby experienced researchers could register for a PhD by publication. For those who might not be altogether familiar with the PhD process, this perhaps requires a little explanation. The usual PhD procedure is to identify an area of research interest, get started on investigating relevant literature, and then gradually identify a particular research problem. Only then would the student be in a position to get started on the actual research investigation that would form the core of the eventual PhD thesis.

The process for a PhD by publication is rather different. One must have already completed a number of research investigations and had accounts of them published before it is possible to have registration for the PhD accepted. These research studies must be linked and related to each other such that they all contribute to the same overall topic or problem area.

In my own case I had, for a number of years, been researching into the experience and performance of our students who were studying on the BA in Applied Social Studies by Independent Study. Carrying out research is a part of the job portfolio of an academic. It seems only appropriate that some of them should research into the other part of the academic job – that is teaching students. Until relatively recently this would not have been seen as a really respectable research area, but this has changed greatly in the last ten to fifteen years. Now there are quite a large number of academic journals which publish research in this area.

My purpose in researching the experience of students and tutors within an independent study degree was to provide a critical examination of the innovative teaching and learning approaches that we used. Most teachers at all levels of the educational system are keen to improve the effectiveness of their teaching. Indeed, these days, this is a professional requirement of the job. A more formal research evaluation can lead to the proposal of teaching improvements. Those possible improvements are then tried out, and evaluated through further research to find out whether they work in practice.

This kind of research approach is different from the traditional expectation that a social researcher should be an objective and unbiased outsider. There are, of course, problems and challenges in being an involved 'action researcher'. Counterbalancing advantages exist in the much more detailed knowledge that the 'insider' researcher will have of the research situation. All the research studies I completed had a focus on improving teaching and student learning within the independent study degree.

The title of my thesis was 'An Evaluation of Teaching and Learning within an Independent Study Degree and Examination of Wider Relevance'. In addition to the inclusion of published research studies, a PhD by publication has to provide an extended, retrospective review. This must place the published studies in a critical context, and explains how the thesis makes both a coherent and significant contribution to knowledge.

I found the writing of this contextual review component of the thesis to be quite a challenging enterprise – more so than I had expected when I started out. At the same time, I found the challenge to be thoroughly absorbing. Both at the time and retrospectively this, for me, was a most satisfying project. One of the benefits of completing a substantial part of the thesis after I had retired was the relaxation of pressure. Alongside the hard work, I was able to take pleasure in what I was doing. The completion of the thesis was a good way of bringing to a conclusion my involvement in independent study over the previous twenty years or so. My PhD was awarded in June 2002. I felt, and still do feel, really pleased with my achievement. For me, it provided a very satisfying culmination to my teaching career.

Being Without a Job...

After the award of the PhD a number of friends made comments along the lines of, 'I bet you are glad to have got that finished and out of the way'. But it wasn't quite like that. As indicated, I was certainly very pleased to have achieved the degree. On the other hand its completion left quite a large gap. I had certainly being doing plenty of other things alongside working on the thesis. However, it had in many ways provided a major framework in my 'working' life. It had constituted an important personal project. In addition it involved an ongoing series of intermediate goals with important opportunities for reward and celebration along the way.

Another loss was that the completion of the thesis reduced my connections with the faculty and university. Though no longer a tutor, I had been a PhD student. As with all PhD students I had regular meetings with my supervisor. These meetings, together with visits to the library, gave me a chance to meet up with my former colleagues. With the PhD completed there was no longer the same requirement for these. I began to feel that the campus was not 'my place' any longer. Now I am a visitor rather than belonging in any kind of way.

So, what is it like and what are the advantages and disadvantages of being without employment, when you have always been used to being in employment? I have in the past, that is when I was still in work, had some cause to investigate the psychological literature on employment. A student whom I supervised had completed an independent project which examined the psychological consequences of unemployment. One important contribution on which she drew was the work of Peter Warr.[1]

Warr had written (in 1987) a still influential book called *Work, Unemployment and Mental Health*. In this book he developed a model which identifies various features, or characteristics of the work environment. He also makes proposals about implications for psychological well-being. Warr suggests that there are a total of nine such factors which have an impact on our lives in employment and beyond. These include the more objective and perhaps most obvious ones of monetary reward and physical safety and security, but also the social position and recognition that derives from that particular job. Other more psychologically oriented aspects of the job context are also identified. He suggests that the extent of the control we have in the job situation, the clarity of the work environment, and whether we know what is expected of us are important aspects. In addition, the extent to which a worker can make use of his or her skills, the existence of appropriate goals and standards, opportunity for inter-personal contact, and the existence of job variety are also important variables.

Warr proposes that for the first three factors outlined above, the more one has of them the better. That is higher levels (e.g. more money) contribute to higher levels of satisfaction. The other aspects also link with and make important contributions to well-being, but only so far. They can be detrimental to well-being at higher levels. For example a degree of variety can make a very important contribution to the interest of a job. On the other hand, too much variety can mean that one constantly has to change from one thing to another, never having an opportunity to get settled with any one task. This is likely to be frustrating and disrupt mental equanimity. Lucky is the person who has all these various job influences at the right level for them!

But what then of the situation where you don't have a job? Do these kinds of factors still have an impact and do they affect well-being and quality of life? Warr's book investigated the effects of unemployment on mental health. The consensus from research findings is that job loss is likely to have a negative influence on personal well being. During unemployment there will tend to be reduced possibilities for control, skill use, social contact etc, as well as less available money and reduced social status.

In contrast with unemployment, many people look forward to retirement. It is one of the normal life transitions. However, for most it will involve some degree of loss and require some readjustments. Retirement as a consequence of ill-health, shares some of the characteristics of 'normal' retirement, but also some of those of un-chosen and unexpected unemployment. Therefore it perhaps requires a greater degree of adjustment. It is not surprising if there are stronger feelings of loss in this kind of situation. So, what are the challenges of being a person with a chronic illness but without a job?

An Alternative Portfolio...

One of the challenges of 'ordinary' retirement is finding satisfying replacement activities to take up the time previously spent in full-time employment. This is certainly a challenge which is shared if one's job is lost as a consequence of becoming ill, or disabled. Also, there may be greater restrictions in terms of what is possible. I certainly cannot fulfil my earlier retirement expectation of taking long walks in the countryside.

With the completion of the PhD there was something of a 'gap' to fill. For some people retirement will provide the opportunity to develop and spend more time on hobbies which they already have. For myself, I cannot say that I already had a well-developed 'hobby-life'. As I've already explained most of my previous spare-time activities were active ones – walking, cycling, skiing – which provided a useful contrast to the relatively sedentary academic life. To a considerable degree these activities were no longer fully available. I needed some new replacement interests. Ideally though I wanted to keep some continuity with my previous life – complete abandonment of what is comfortably familiar is probably not sensible.

So, what kind of alternative portfolio is developing? First of all, what are the interests that I can keep going? I am still a psychologist – even if now in a private capacity. I keep up with reading in the area – although with slightly adjusted areas of interest. Much of this is now focused loosely around the business of adjusting to, and coping with chronic illness. I am also exploring the newly emerging area of positive psychology. The other continuing activity that helps to keep me busy is writing. A major occupation has been writing this book. From time to time, I am also involved in writing much smaller scale pieces.

To a degree, the new interests I am developing have also emerged out of past ones. In my second year at grammar school I had to abandon the study of history as I wanted to continue with science subjects. As I've indicated, I wasn't very pleased about that, for I was interested in history as well as science. Now, I have the opportunity to take up this interest again. I have only just begun and am really only 'looking around' this new (for me) discipline. There are so many possibilities, in terms of aspects and periods to investigate, and so many good books. There is plenty here to absorb my interest.

My education has also been somewhat deficient linguistically. I do not speak a foreign language with any degree of fluency. I passed an O level in German, but that was 40 years ago and, despite some periodic revision efforts, I can't really carry on a proper conversation.

I had thoughts of trying to improve my German, but instead I've decided to move in a different linguistic direction. When I was in the sixth form I got interested in the international language Esperanto, as it seemed such a sensible idea. I got as far as buying *Teach Yourself Esperanto,* but not much further. An article in the *Guardian* newspaper rekindled my interest and so I have embarked on learning Esperanto.

The other pastime that I am intending to cultivate, though I haven't progressed very far, is a creative one. I would like to draw, and maybe paint a little. This is an entirely new departure and one in which I don't think I have any native talent – but I would like to explore the possibilities.

A Motivational Landscape…

How is this new (and renewed) portfolio of interests going to work? Will they keep me busy and satisfied? Will they be enjoyable? Or are they too serious and academic? To some extent time will tell. But in the meantime I think that there are some contributions from the psychological literature which might help in contemplating and assessing the possibilities. These contributions come in terms of ideas about serious leisure, flow and personal projects. These concepts have the potential to contribute to our understanding of the motivational landscape through which our lives are mapped out. They are not at odds with our ordinary, everyday understanding, but perhaps a more refined map and guide can offer additional insights.

The idea of 'serious' leisure might appear rather contradictory. After all, leisure is for fun and enjoyment isn't it? Yes, but maybe it is for more than that! Robert Stebbins has argued that leisure can usefully be viewed as a serious matter.[2] He proposes that serious leisure requires time and effort. It is also likely to require the acquisition of new knowledge and special skills. Stebbins suggests that it can extend to almost embarking on an alternative career and perhaps entering a new social grouping of fellow practitioners.

One form of serious leisure which Stebbins identifies is that of a serious amateur interest. This involves taking up for leisure purposes some pursuit which also constitutes a professional occupation. An example would be someone who is an amateur astronomer, or an amateur historian. A variant on the theme of serious leisure is someone who is a devoted hobbyist. The builder and tinkerer with models or machines would fall into this category. The liberal arts hobbyist is another kind of enthusiast who is concerned with the systematic acquisition of knowledge for its own sake accomplished through voracious reading.

So, what are the benefits? Important rewards come, for example, through a sense of achievement, of satisfaction, personal enrichment and social solidarity with fellow practitioners. On the other hand, just because the interest is being taken seriously, there is also the potential for costs such as failures and disappointment, and interpersonal conflict with fellow practitioners. For those who continue their investment in their serious leisure pursuit the rewards obviously outweigh the costs.

The idea of 'flow', which has developed through the work of Mihaly Csikszentmihalyi,[3] has some common ground with serious leisure, but also provides a slightly different 'slant' on possible alternative activities. So, what *is* flow? In what kind of circumstances is it likely to be generated? I think that the best way to gain an understanding is in terms of an example. One relevant practice which Csikszentmihalyi has investigated is that of rock climbing. As non-climbers, we perhaps wonder why people get involved in this obviously dangerous pasttime. But, maybe, thinking in terms of flow can give us some appreciation of the attraction.

Most of us would agree that rock climbing is rather a challenging business. You are going to have to concentrate pretty hard. You need a considerable degree of skill to even think about getting up there. It is also crucial that the climb you have chosen matches appropriately to your skill level. You want it to be challenging – but not too challenging! When you climb you are obviously going to be paying very close attention to what you are doing – concentration doesn't and cannot lapse. You are completely absorbed in the challenge of the climb.

These kinds of responses and this kind of experience epitomise flow. We are likely to experience flow when we are engaged on some task or activity that requires skill and effort, is challenging, but is just within our capabilities. Such engagement means that we get engrossed in the present moment, in what we are doing. Self-consciousness disappears; time seems to stop, or rather passes with us hardly being aware that it is doing so.

Of course, rock climbing is just one of many activities or preoccupations which can generate flow. There are many physical activities and skills that will do so. For me, in the past, skiing has certainly been one of these. Artistic practices have also been investigated in this connection and already I can see that my very limited attempts at drawing provide the possibility of flow experiences.

I have more substantial experience of achieving a sense of flow through writing. At the same time my experience suggests that it is easy to exaggerate the extent and universality of flow during those activities and practices which ought to be conducive to its emergence. To continue the 'flow' metaphor, flows can get diverted, come up against rocky obstacles, or sink into deep pools. In my experience of writing, positive flow can similarly lose its impetus or dry up altogether. Serious effort is required to maintain progress. But difficulties overcome do lead to satisfaction.

Thus, it is being argued that these kinds of activities (including at least some that are products of serious leisure) are rewarding and satisfying in and of themselves. There is a sense in which they are enjoyable although this is not the focus of our engagement. Rather it is something that we feel as we look back on our achievement and the task, which was previously taking the whole of our attention.

Both serious leisure and flow generating experiences provide a basis for continuing areas of interest. Once started, they are quite likely to be sustained for a substantial period – they provide ongoing pre-occupations. However, within these continuing interests we are also likely to have more specific goals and projects. My third contributor to marking out the motivational landscape, Brian Little, has focused specifically on the personal projects which he suggests most of us have.[4]

Little has investigated people's personal projects by asking them to identify those that are currently important. Respondents do not usually find it difficult to identify a list of such projects of varying 'weights', significance and expected duration. A few of my current projects are to get to the end of my present set of Esperanto lessons, to drive a bit more, to keep up and extend my meditation practice, to plan and organise our next holiday. These projects are likely to be personal and idiosyncratic in character reflecting the various tasks and interests that are part of our lives.

As well as being concerned to identify people's varied and idiosyncratic projects, Little is interested in how they are proceeding and working out. He has asked respondents about this in terms of a number of dimensions such as enjoyment, importance, challenge, difficulty, control and outcome. He has also examined the temporal stages in terms of which we initiate, implement, complete – or withdraw from projects.

I am currently finding my overall 'Esperanto project' perhaps a little more difficult than I had expected. I had thought the whole point of the international language was that it should be easy to learn! Well, yes…but up to a point. I have a good distance learning course, and a tutor who gives prompt and positive feedback (*Bona respondaro,* or even *bonege*). But, as he points out, learning any language requires considerable sustained effort. There certainly are difficult bits. Also, acquiring oral proficiency in Esperanto has its problems – there aren't people immediately around to talk to. I am certainly finding having phone conversations with my tutor in Esperanto rather challenging at the moment!

So, at any one time, it is likely that some of our projects will be progressing well, others less so. We may be on the verge of suspending, or trying to disengage from the one that is really posing problems, but celebrating a degree of success in another. Little suggests that they can be represented as an intersecting lattice of possibilities, deriving from recreational interests, maybe employment requirements, and the multifaceted demands of ordinary life. In overall terms, he has presented evidence to suggest that life satisfaction has some links with the general ease and efficacy with which we negotiate our personal projects. Thus, as well as identifying individual interests and projects to keep us busy, we need to try and manage the whole portfolio of possibilities in a way that is as fulfilling as possible.

Days in a Life…

So how is the set of interests and activities that *I* have developed progressing? How do things work out on a day to day basis and in the longer term? To what extent does my portfolio of possibilities provide a satisfying alternative to the job which I gave up? I think that the answer is probably positive – on the whole.

The first thing to be said is that I feel busy and occupied through the day. I often still feel that I don't have time to do everything I want to. I do have a rough and ready plan for what I want to accomplish during the day, and perhaps over the week, but deadlines are much less significant. To a considerable extent tasks emerge out of, or are prompted by, the framework and routine that I have established for myself.

I do some writing most days. Sometimes this goes well, and I feel that I have achieved something useful, but, of course, there are times when less progress is made. Quite often there is something to read, or look up, which is associated with that writing, so that is a different kind of activity. Currently, another constituent of my day is working on my Esperanto course. Some days I will do some Esperanto as well as the writing. Otherwise I will be concentrating on just one of these. Singly, or together, these will take up several hours of most weekdays.

A different kind of enjoyment comes from getting out and about, which I do most days. I feel particularly lucky that I can take advantage of a beautiful day – either by having a ride on my trike, or a walk down the lane. Actually, it is fine and pleasant enough to get out most days now that I can choose my time. I also usually take some indoors exercise. I have my short exercise session first thing. If I'm not having a walk I try to have a reasonably vigorous (but short) 'hop' to some appropriate music. Then there is the early evening yoga 'spot' when Pete usually joins in.

These days, I can't really avoid at least some of the household chores. When I worked, and for a while afterwards, someone else did the cleaning. But now our long-term cleaner has moved on to a different kind of job and I have had to 'knuckle down' to the work, or parts of it. Many of the chores I can do. The strategy has to be to do a little at a time. This is partly because I get tired if I do too much – frustratingly I can get tired from just standing up for too long – but also to keep motivated.

So, with a few other additions, the days are filled easily and busily. There is enough variety in what I can do during the day to keep me interested and involved. I achieve sufficient to provide a sense of positive accomplishment over the day. I also have a degree of freedom and choice about what to do – probably more so than when I was in work. I can take control of my day and make my own decisions. In terms of Warr's model of the environmental working conditions, which promote well-being, I am probably doing quite well.

But there is also a need to keep an appropriate balance in relation to some aspects. Most obviously I need to manage my physical activities, and especially their aftermath appropriately. These are important and valuable to me but they make me tired – usually when I get home from a walk or ride it is quite impossible to do anything more. First, I need to keep the sense of frustration which can easily arise within bounds; secondly, I ideally should have planned something else to do which doesn't require any expenditure of energy.

The other kind of balance relates to the self set goals. Retirement clearly provides the possibility of 'sitting back', relaxing and taking things easy. However, the contributors whose ideas were reviewed earlier in this chapter would take a different position. Their underlying message is that we need to accept challenges and put in effort in order to obtain satisfaction and reward. On the other hand I know that if I am aiming too high, achieving a feeling of success and appropriate self reinforcement is going to be more difficult. Being chronically ill, with reduced energy and capability, means that it is not easy to achieve as much as I used to. It is hard to accept this and negotiate changed expectations.

Another change which I am facing as a consequence of leaving work is the absence of work colleagues. In work it is easy to take these people for granted, but they provide a ready source of comfortable social contact. Because you are working together, on the same job, there are plenty of things to talk about. I have now chosen, at least for the time being, to fill my day with relatively solitary activities. I am also conscious that psychologists have suggested that a well-developed social network is supportive of well-being. I do miss, to a degree, the social and intellectual 'buzz' of meeting with colleagues and students. However, I am very much an introvert – I am largely happy with my own company for much of the day. I am, of course, not on my own all the time. I often meet neighbours when I am out; I meet ex-colleagues periodically at the university; I have Pete's company during the evening; and, of course, we continue to arrange social activities with friends. So, it is by no means entirely a solitary existence!

The Best Decision?

Clearly, I have not fulfilled my original hope, in the early days of my MS, that I might be able to stay in my lecturing post. I was inspired by the example of Charles Evans, but I decided not to follow in his footsteps. So, was leaving my job the right decision – or was it some kind of defeat?

As I've already indicated, the decision to stay in employment or not is one of the most difficult and complex ones to be faced by anybody who becomes chronically ill and disabled. Overall, I think that the decision to leave work was the most appropriate, for I have been able to find other things with which to fill my time. The life of Sir Charles Evans still inspires me, but in facing a life with chronic illness and disability I have realised that it is crucial to make my own decisions, and take the path I have chosen for myself, rather than thinking of emulating others.

There is also a recognition that I have been hugely fortunate in the extent of the difficulties that I have faced. I became ill and disabled relatively late in life after achieving most things that were important to me within my career. Of course there have been financial penalties, but these have been moderate rather than severe. I am very well aware that employment difficulties are much more problematic for many people who become disabled in mid career, and especially if family responsibilities are high.

Currently, there is a great deal of pressure on individuals who find themselves in this situation to stay in, or return to, work. That pressure is both financial and moral in character. The present *zeitgeist* would seem to be that if it is at all possible one ought to be working. Certainly, there are many important ways in which the employment situation for people with disabilities has improved over recent years. Today there are legal requirements for the support and protection of disabled workers which are helpful to a degree.

However, there have been other changes in the work situation which have counteracted these legislative improvements. It is undoubtedly the case that the pace and pressures of the work situation have increased over recent years for everybody. Because of this there is much discussion of the difficulties able bodied people have in maintaining an appropriate work-life balance. As Susan Wendell has pointed out in some detail, this increased pace and pressure means that it has become impossible for many people with disabilities to cope with the kind of full time jobs which in previous times they would have been able to manage.[5] But being forced into a part time mode can bring with it obvious financial penalties.

The difficulties of providing an appropriate employment framework for people with disabilities are considerable, and are certainly quite a long way from being resolved.

Notes and References

1. Warr, P. (1987). *Work, Unemployment, and Mental Health*. Oxford: Clarendon Press.

2. An accessible article on serious leisure (Serious leisure and well-being) by Stebbins is available in Haworth, J. T. (1997). *Work, Leisure and Well-being*. London: Routledge.

3. An edited examination of issues related to flow is provided in Csikszentmihlyi, M. & Csikszentmihalyi, I. S. (1988) (Eds.). *Optimal experience: Psychological studies of flow in consciousness*. Cambridge: Cambridge University Press.

4. An accessible account of Little's ideas is found in one of his earlier articles. Little, B. R. (1983). Personal projects: A rationale and method for investigation. *Environment and Behaviour*, 15 (3), 273-309.

5. Discussed in Wendell, S. (1996). *The Rejected Body*. New York: Routledge. pp. 37-39.

Chapter Eight

Cycling Differently

Cycling was an important part of our lives prior to my getting MS. After our return from our Bavarian cycling holiday, and then the huge shock of the MS diagnosis in September 1993, I didn't know whether I would ever be able to cycle again. I didn't have the courage to try getting back on my bike, as my walking balance was so bad it wasn't worth the risk. I was worried not only about physical injury if I fell off, but also the feelings of disappointment and upset that were sure to result if I found that I couldn't cycle.

Previously, cycling had been such an important contribution to keeping fit. If cycling outside in the conventional way was going to be a bit risky, I wondered whether cycling inside, on a stationary bike might be the next best option. We bought some cycle rollers, Pete set these up in the garage and my bike was transformed into an exercise bike! I started cycling inside.

It was good to be 'on the bike again' so to speak. It helped a great deal to have a cyclometer so I could easily check my speed and distance and set targets. To begin with I was doing one or two miles, but before too long I could sometimes manage up to four miles. This was about the maximum I could manage physically, but also before boredom really set in. I soon discovered that this kind of cycling is really boring. Most of the enjoyment of cycling, for me at least, comes from being outside and going somewhere and having the stimulus of changing scenery.

It wasn't too long therefore before I decided that I must take the risk and give proper outside cycling another try. On a Sunday, just after the beginning of November 1993, we took the bike off the rollers and outside onto the drive. I got on as carefully as I could – but it was OK – no real problem. We set off 'round the block'. Pete was running alongside in case I looked as though I was falling off, but everything went well. We only did half a mile, but I felt hugely pleased and that this was a really great achievement – I was back on my bike – properly!

Over the succeeding months we gradually extended that half mile substantially. By the middle of 1994, I had achieved rides of around seven to eight miles, a terrific boost to morale. In many ways, especially in those early months of recovery, cycling was easier than walking. It felt more co-ordinated, more like it should do, and less tiring. We had regular outings into the local South Cheshire lanes. I felt very lucky that we could so easily get out into pleasant cycling country.

By the summer of 1995 I was feeling more and more confident about my cycling abilities and stamina and we decided to try a cycling weekend away from home. We didn't feel up to proper touring but instead chose a fixed base with plans for day tours. We stayed at a small guest house on the southern coast of Anglesey, beyond Beaumaris. It was a lovely peaceful spot with views over the Menai straits towards the mountains of Snowdonia.

It was a very successful weekend. We were lucky with the weather. We explored the quiet back roads of the island – some hills but not too many. It felt a great achievement when I completed a total of 19 miles over one of the days. That is not much of a total for a serious cyclist, but then we had never been ones to pile on the miles. We had always preferred a reasonably relaxed pace with plenty of stops for exploration off the bikes. It was good to feel that, at least in this respect, we were pretty well back to a pre-MS level of operation.

Another Continental Holiday…

Emboldened by the success of the Anglesey weekend, we planned another cycling holiday in Europe – just two years after our Bavarian holiday and the beginnings of my MS. We chose the kind of holiday that was similar to the ones we had taken previously, the lazy way of doing things. It is cycle touring where the holiday firm does the hard work of organising a route, and finding and booking comfortable hotels for overnight stays.

At the end of July we set off in our car for the Burgundy area of France. We had picked one of the easiest, least strenuous tours. It involved a circular route that began at the tiny village of Cravant on the banks of the river Yonne. Our first day of cycling was along a riverside road and then along the tow path as the river was canalised. This took us to the attractive town of Auxerre with interesting old churches and timber framed houses. Then a day to explore, since the procedure for the holiday was one day of cycling followed by a 'rest' day if you wished, or a day cycling tour if you were keen to stay 'on the bike'. In other words, we stayed for two nights at our hotel in Auxerre.

After that we headed into the depths of the French countryside, through gently rolling countryside and attractive villages. It was easy cycling. Our destination the next night was the medium sized village (a main street with a few small shops) of Ligny-le-Chatel. Our hotel was on this main street, entered through an archway, into an attractive courtyard which gave access to some of the rooms, including ours. The main part of the hotel, with dining room, was immediately off the street. We explored the village in the late afternoon and were just in time to get into an interesting art exhibition in the village hall.

The next day, we did cycle on our 'rest day' having mapped out a fairly easy and not overlong route of about 16 miles. This compared with the usual tour mileage of around 20 to 25 miles, which I was relieved and pleased to find that I was managing without any problem.

From Ligny the route was back to base at Cravant. In some ways this was perhaps the most attractive day's cycling. The initial part of the ride was on a very quiet riverside road, passing through a couple of small villages. Then we reached the larger village of Chablis, the centre of the famous wine growing area. Since we had a fair amount of cycling still to do we decided not to indulge, but instead we sat in the cafe in the middle of the village square and succumbed to a large, multi-flavoured sorbet with extra fruit and fruit sauce.

The latter part of the day's route initially required a greater degree of effort, a long, slow pedal uphill, but worth it for the beautiful and extensive views over the rolling hills and valleys covered with vineyards. Then, of course, we had the reward of a long downhill swoop, back into the village of Cravant.

It is always sad when a holiday comes to an end, but in many ways I felt like celebrating this ending. I was so pleased that it had all been so enjoyable and successful; I had managed the cycling without any kind of problem, and now I was optimistic that cycling possibilities were again opening up, although I still knew that they might not last.

Balance problems…

Quite soon, unfortunately, things did change As we entered into the autumn of 1995 my physical capability, mentioned earlier, began to slowly decline. At first it was my walking that was most affected. My cycling legs kept going rather longer. I don't know why but somehow or other the cycling movement didn't seem to tire me out quite so much as walking. But I did get tired and we were reduced to doing shorter local rides.

At the beginning of March 1996, I realised that I was having some difficulty getting on to my bike. As one part of this relapse, my balance was deteriorating badly. Balance is obviously an important requirement in the cycling business, particularly as you are getting onto the bike and especially with a diamond frame. You have to balance on one leg while swinging the other over the bar. I could feel that I was getting less secure as I did this.

The crisis came later that month. We had been out for a local ride of around three to four miles, and within a half mile or so of home my legs became so tired that I knew I had to have a rest. The problem was that I was so tired that I couldn't get off the bike in the usual way – the balance required was impossible. It was all over so quickly that it is hard to say what actually happened. My best recollection is that I had a fairly controlled fall into the bank at the side of the road. Fortunately Pete was there to disentangle me from the bike. He could also get home easily to fetch the car and come and pick me up. Quite suddenly, the option of getting out on my bike had gone. Freedom was lost. It was very hard to accept being limited and restricted in this way so soon after that marvellous holiday, when my hopes had been so high.

A Custom Built Trike….

So, we were back to the situation where the only way I could cycle was inside on the rollers. Here, of course, balance wasn't an issue, so I could keep cycling. Stamina was a problem, but then I could stop whenever I needed to. I tried hard to keep up my enthusiasm for roller cycling!

But, it was never the same. I wanted to be out there, on the road, in the open air. A new way had to be found so I could cycle again. We soon realised the obvious option was to acquire a tricycle! I could ride as slowly as I wanted and there would be no problem in relation to balance. Conveniently, one of the best tricycle builders in the country, George Longstaff, had his shop and workshop not far from where we live.

We delayed and dithered for a little while as we tried to decide between a trike and a tandem trike. The latter are very attractive machines. There would be the advantage that since both of us would be riding together on the same trike, I could 'borrow' some power from Pete. My lack of stamina would be less of a limitation. However, there would be a disadvantage – I couldn't go out cycling on my own. For me this was quite an important consideration – I wanted to have the option of cycling by myself even if I wasn't able to get that far.

I decided in favour of the tricycle for one. We visited George Longstaff and discussed my needs and preferences. George has a long-standing interest in, and experience of, catering for the needs of disabled cyclists. Tandem trikes, for example, have particular advantages for rear, 'stoker' riders who have sight problems. The little luxury we chose for my trike was a rear differential which would allow me to turn the trike around within a small turning circle. Thus, if I was reaching the end of my energy while cycling along a narrow lane, I would be able to turn around without any difficulty.

Fortunately for George, he is a busy man, with a full order book for custom built bikes and trikes. So, I needed a degree of patience. We ordered the trike in the late Spring of 1996 and took delivery in the September. It was, and is, to my eyes a splendid machine. We had decided on a dark green paint job. George Longstaff's name is there in gold lettering on the ascending tube of the frame. It is a name that is recognised by committed cyclists and we have often found ourselves exchanging reminiscences about George, or discussing the merits of tricycle riding.

Non-tricycle riders, essentially the great majority of the population, will be unaware that the transfer from riding a bike to a trike has its difficulties. On a bike one is continually, and automatically, correcting for the tendency of the bike to fall over. On a trike this is obviously not required. You have to get used to not correcting. To begin with it means that the trike has a tendency to steer down the camber and into the left gutter. There is a need to accommodate to this – initially consciously and deliberately – though it soon becomes automatic.

I soon overcame these little challenges and began to really enjoy the short rides I took along the local lanes. However, my joy did not last long. The MS was now affecting leg power and soon I was getting muscle spasms in my left leg when I was working it too hard – which really wasn't very hard at all

So, the pleasure I had expected to get from the trike was curtailed. By the early weeks of 1997 I had given up. I had found that after only a mile or two of cycling, the spasms in my leg, often jerking my leg off the pedal, were becoming really annoying and frustrating. I just couldn't control my leg and stop it going into spasm. I lost patience – I couldn't enjoy the experience any more.

This was yet another major upset. I had felt so pleased with my new tricycle – it was beautiful, elegant and special. The trike had given me the ability to get around easily and conveniently, which I could no longer get from walking, and I had so enjoyed getting out and riding around. It came very hard to lose this freedom almost immediately after I had discovered it

However, there was still some optimism lurking under the huge disappointment. You never know what will happen – good or bad – with MS. My wonderful tricycle had to be relegated to the garage – but I couldn't bring myself to sell it.

Handcycle Discovery…

What else could I do to keep mobile, and get actively out and about? At the end of 1997 the cycling scene changed again. I came upon a completely new possibility. I found out about *hand*cycles. At the Crewe+Alsager Faculty of Manchester Metropolitan University where I still worked, there is a well established and highly regarded

Department of Sport and Exercise Science. Within the department there is an interest in sport for people with disabilities. As part of their course provision the department has put on a BA in Sport and Disability. One of my colleagues in this department passed on to me some literature about handcycling. This was a great help as there is not a huge amount of publicity about these machines. It would certainly have taken me longer to discover them without this tip, in fact, I could quite easily not have found out at all!

What *is* a handcycle? How does it work? To some degree the name is self-explanatory. One cycles using hands and arms rather than feet and legs. But how is this done? What kind of machine makes it possible?

My handcycle is an attachment to my wheelchair (Handcycles are also available in purpose built form.) It comprises a single wheel with attached frame, chain wheels providing 21 speed derrailleur gears and handlebars, which together provide the front end of the handcycle. This front end is attached to the wheelchair, via an under seat socket, to make up the complete handcycle which is effectively a different kind of tricycle. The handlebars are cranked in a circular, push – pull movement of both arms to provide forward motion for the whole machine. Both arms work together unlike normal cycling where the legs work alternatively. Both arms together provide a stronger push – pull force.

It took a little while to decide to investigate the handcycling option. Taking this path involved acceptance that proper cycling was no longer likely to be possible, but before long I decided that a rather different form of cycling was much better than no cycling. If I was going to stay physically active, a readiness to experiment and be flexible was necessary.

We travelled to Liverpool to investigate Chevron Wheelchairs who also manufacture 'add on' handcycles. Their workshop is situated on a dockside industrial estate not far from Albert Dock. Here we met

Vince Ross, who is a crucial member of the firm. Vince is a paraplegic, as a result of an accident, and a handcycling enthusiast, as well as a manufacturer of these machines. He talked of heading off for the Lake District with the handcycle in the back of his estate car and of taking part, with other handcyclists, in a recent Chester to Liverpool charity cycle ride. Clearly, there were all sorts of possibilities here.

Vince soon organised a machine that I could try out for myself. There was plenty of largely traffic free space on the estate. It was good to be moving at a reasonable speed again, and as a result of my own active involvement. It was, however, immediately clear that handcycling would demand a fair amount of effort. Vince's comment was, 'I didn't say it was going to be easy'.

Easy or not, we soon decided that a handcycle would open up avenues that would otherwise be closed, and ordered the 'front end' handcycle which would fit onto my existing wheelchair. It would be in bright yellow to match the chair. First though, the wheelchair needed some modification. The chair folds for easier transport and storage, but, as Vince put it, you don't want to be doing 30 mph down a hill when the chair starts to collapse. So, it had to be strengthened and the fitting of the socket added for the joining up of the handcycle part of the combined machine.

These modifications were quickly completed, and we collected the reconditioned wheelchair and new handcycle addition towards the end of March 1998. Generally it takes a while to get used to using a new piece of exercise equipment, but a handcycle doesn't require too much in terms of skill acquisition. However it does require increased arm strength and stamina, which are only acquired slowly. I found that the majority of handcyclists are, like Vince, male paraplegics. They have two advantages: being male they have greater arm strength to begin with, and, as paraplegics, they use their arms rather more than I do.

Initially, I had assumed that the handcycle would be a bicycle replacement. Pete would be on his bike and I would handcycle alongside (or behind, or in front, as conditions dictated). However, I soon discovered that I couldn't really go fast enough – unless it was downhill. Trying to handcycle up any kind of serious hill was a major frustration – almost a total impossibility. I would come to a standstill on even quite minor hills, even in the lowest gear!

Fortunately, alongside these impediments, there were also positive experiences. Soon after acquiring the handcycle, towards the end of May 1998, we joined my parents and sister on a week's holiday in Pembrokeshire. Here, using the handcycle was a very positive experience – but I was handcycling when the others were walking. We didn't go any great distances. My parents are in their eighties and my father has arthritic knees so the walks were only short ones of a couple of miles or so. Nevertheless, this was more than I could have done if I'd been walking.

So, on the basis of this and our other early experience with the handcycle, I soon came to the conclusion that handcycling provided a better 'walking replacement' than the electric 'buggy'. There were a number of reasons for this judgement. First of all, using the handcycle is very much an active process, whereas using the buggy largely involves merely sitting there and steering. There are more positive feelings of satisfaction when doing something for and by myself.

I do, though, accept help when it is useful, and a second advantage of the handcycle is that it is much lighter than the electric buggy. An able bodied companion can therefore assist with 'push power' on short steep sections, or 'lifting power' over minor obstacles. The handcycle can also be taken apart into its two main parts, and, if necessary, the wheels taken off the wheelchair section. In this way we can, on occasion manage to get it over stiles and such like. With this greater flexibility the challenge of seeing where we can get to becomes a much more enjoyable, rewarding and interesting one.

The third value of handcycling as against riding the buggy is that handcycling provides excellent exercise. You may not be using your legs, but you are certainly using your arms. Climbing any kind of incline is hard work and makes serious demands in terms of heart activity.

It is probably clear that the handcycle has proved a major success. It is possible to use the handcycle over reasonably rough ground. In some ways I use the handcycle as a mountain bike equivalent, but my companion is walking rather than cycling.

Many of our previous walking haunts are no longer accessible. However, it is surprising where you can get to once you start investigating. Country Parks, canal side paths, old railway trails and forestry routes provide obvious possibilities. Other recent, perhaps more surprising excursions have been on parts of the coastal path in Pembrokeshire, getting half way up Snowdon on the Miners track and over the salt flats on the north Norfolk coast. Courtesy of the handcycle I can still get to beautiful places.

Tricycling Again…

But I still wasn't able to do any 'proper' on-road cycling, although I had managed to get back to garage roller cycling from November 1998. I'm not quite sure why this hadn't prompted me to try out the tricycle again. I presume it was because I was getting started on the handcycling enterprise and was thinking that this was now the best way forward for my future cycling.

However, in April 1999 I did have new thoughts about retrying the tricycle, prompted by an advert I saw in the *On Your Bike* magazine from The Electric Bike Company. They were promoting the advantages of battery supported motorised cycling which led me to wonder if I might be able to ride my tricycle again if I had a bit of power assistance. I phoned up the *Electric Bike* people to ask them to send some information.

Before I got too hopeful it seemed sensible to have a short trial with the tricycle. I got on rather carefully. This felt better than the last time I had tried. I set off round the block, which was a distance of around half a mile, and accomplished this without any sign of leg spasms. Thus encouraged, I tried a distance more like a proper ride. When I did three miles without any problems I really began to feel that cycling might be possible again. Then over the May Bank Holiday I completed distances of around five miles on each of two successive days. I was overjoyed and could hardly believe it was happening. I was ready to try battery supported cycling!

In the meantime, information had arrived from the electric bike company. The most suitable (but also most expensive) appeared to be the Heinzmann Power Hub. This would involve building a new front wheel to include the electrically powered hub motor and then linking this up to a nickel cadmium battery fixed onto the rear carrier.

Next there was a phone call from Richard Burkinshaw, who is our nearest representative of the *Electric Bike* network, based at Brighouse in Yorkshire. We had a useful, not too technical discussion about speeds, weights, hill climbing power, battery range and recharging. Richard offers to collect the owner's bike (or trike!) for fitting and then returns it after modification. Also, the company has a policy of refunding the money within 30 days if the purchaser is not satisfied. It began to feel this was something I had to try.

Further investigation was undertaken by going up to Brighouse to see the machines, though I couldn't actually have a trial run since there weren't any powered up trikes available. Given my problems with balance I didn't think that it would be sensible to risk life and limb on an ordinary bike. Pete had a quick spin on a sample machine and reported favourably. The decision was made and the tricycle left behind for modification that Saturday.

Fortunately, I didn't have to wait long to get it back. It was delivered to our house, all set up with hub motor, battery and twist grip control system on the following Thursday – excellent service. After a brief discussion over keys and switches and batteries, I had a quick initial trial run around the block. This was a flat run, so not a serious trial, but all the new equipment seemed easy to use. In spite of the extra weight of motor and battery, riding without power didn't seem that much more effort than previously.

Soon the powered-up trike was properly put through its paces and I had got accustomed to using it. When feeling strong, I can use the trike in the normal way without any power assistance. When I'm tired, or have a hill to climb, I can 'add in' an appropriate amount of power assistance. It is also possible to ride with power support without any pedalling. I mostly do this to start up in awkward spots which would otherwise require a degree of leg and foot pressure which I cannot any longer summon up.

I try to keep the power assistance to a minimum – I usually keep cycling up the hills but with an added boost. The twist grip control is superb and works as the name suggests. After having switched on, the left handlebar grip is turned forwards to access the power – twisting further forward produces greater acceleration. The twist grip is quite sensitive so the tricycle never feels out of control. The battery power lasts for around 25 miles of cycling and there are indicator lights to show when it is running low.

It felt marvellous to have the trike back in commission and whenever I go out I appreciate this anew. I now ride regularly – up to around four times a week. Even in the winter I get out when the weather allows – which is actually quite frequently. Since I can choose when to go out I am usually able to avoid the rain. For most weekday outings I am doing somewhere around four to five miles. I am enormously lucky that I can easily and quickly get out from our house on to quiet back roads. The cycling would be nothing like as pleasant if I was on busy, main ones. I have three local circuits which I can join up in different combinations, which gives me a reasonably varied set of easily accessible routes.

I also ride into town. I have acquired a large, traditional, wicker-work bike basket, useful for the quick dumping of purchases, and in many ways it is better to cycle into town than take the car. It is in line with my environmental convictions and I can feel (somewhat smugly) superior to able-bodied shoppers who have *driven* a mile or two into town. I have to admit though that it is more convenient for me to cycle. Using the tricycle I can cycle around town and stop briefly to make a particular purchase. If I use the car I have to park, then leave it and walk around. This means that I get tired quickly and there is a greater limitation in the distance I can go and the shopping stops that I can make.

So, I'm now doing quite a bit of tricycling. Acquiring the tricycle has, after all, proved to be well worth while. As well as riding locally, I often ride a little bit further with Pete at weekends. During the holiday periods we also manage longer rides in other parts of the country. Overall, I've been completing somewhere around 1,000 miles a year.

Tandem Trials…

As I've said, Pete had earlier suggested that getting a tandem tricycle would be a good way for us to continue cycling. I had resisted because I wanted the option of going out on my own. However, at the beginning of 2002 we began to think further about tandem possibilities. Since I had been able to ride my tricycle again, Pete and I had enjoyed cycling together at weekends and holiday time. But our cycling capabilities were still not fully matched. Pete has to cycle relatively slowly to keep pace with me. A suitable tandem set-up would allow the two of us to combine effort – or for me to benefit from Pete's greater strength and stamina, and could provide a better experience of cycling together.

The most obvious strategy was to ask George Longstaff to build us a tandem trike. George is the best (only?) tandem trike builder in the country[1]. As well as constructing purpose built tandems, made to measure for particular customers, George also produces a (somewhat) cheaper version. He buys mass produced tandems, removes the back wheel and replaces it with a new tricycle 'rear end'. George had suggested to us on one or two occasions that he thought we would be able to cycle further on such a machine than I could on my single trike.

However, before we made a positive decision, Pete felt that he needed to investigate other possibilities, in particular to find out whether there was anything suitable in the way of recumbent tandems. It might be thought (and I tended to agree) it was a somewhat esoteric proposal which wouldn't come to much. But we do have some copies of a publication which is full of many and various quite esoteric cycles – this is *Encycleopedia* which reviews amazing cycles for all sorts of purposes from across the world.

A little research did indeed identify two such cycles. The first was the Australian Greenspeed recumbent tandem trike, but with one rider being positioned behind the other it seemed a rather long machine. The other one was the Trice which is a British designed side by side recumbent tandem, with the option of hand cranking on one side.

But, before we got round to visiting, we were off on an Easter holiday to Norfolk – and a different option arose. While we were there, we used a day to drive over to Little Thetford, which is just a few miles from the cathedral city of Ely on the edge of the Fens. The objective of this excursion was to visit D. Tec HPVs – 'The UK's Largest Recumbent Dealer' – selling both new, and also lots of second hand models. Such a visit is an experience in itself. The owner, Kevin, deals from home and his garage and the forecourt of the house are crowded with recumbents in all shapes and sizes. I had no idea that they came in such a huge variety!

After a little while spent viewing the different machines, and after Pete had tried out a one person recumbent or two, we were introduced to the German made Pino. This is an interesting machine, being a relatively short tandem with a recumbent front end. Unusually, the rear rider is the one who is in control and has the handlebars, brakes, gears etc. This rider is seated higher than the front rider and so has the necessary clear forward view. Thus, probably uniquely for a tandem, both riders can see to the front. The other advantage, as it I saw it, was that both riders were seated higher up than is the case with many recumbents.

I was still dubious about it though – I hadn't been on a two wheeled cycle for around five years – but was persuaded to give it a try. So we rode up and down the road outside the D. Tek premises. I wouldn't say I felt that secure but at least we kept upright.

I agreed to a longer trial. For this we had to venture over to the other side of a dual carriageway, a brave move – well for me anyway! Neither of us had ridden a tandem before and I couldn't readily get my feet back on the ground to help in the balancing, as my feet were out in front on the recumbent bit and securely fitted in toe clips. And the dual carriageway was a very busy road – so finding a space in the traffic and then making a quick get away would be no easy matter. Anyway we got across – or rather Pete got us there. My task was the relatively easy one of sitting there and then peddling as fast as possible when the gap came. It was easier on the quieter roads over the other side, although there were still some junctions to negotiate.

But we both enjoyed our ride of five to six miles. It was good to be cycling together. The cycling position on the Pino is a very sociable and companionable one as the heads of both riders are fairly close together and so conversation is easy. I also found that I very much enjoyed the experience of cycling faster than I could on my trike. I was nearly converted.

Another advantage of the Pino is that hand cranks can be substituted for the pedals of the recumbent portion of the tandem. This meant that if my legs and feet ceased to be able to manage the pedals, the purchase of an extra fitting would allow me to move straight into hand cranking, and the whole tandem would not be redundant.

Back home we gave the two options serious thought. Should it be the Pino or a tandem trike? Having worked out the pros and cons of each machine we still found it difficult to decide. We really needed proper comparative trials of both machines.

Luckily, George Longstaff had a tandem trike that would fit us at his workshop. (He doesn't have much of a supply of machines as he normally makes them to customer's order.) He agreed to lend it to us for a weekend trial. This was, on all counts, amazingly successful. He had been right about the distance I would be able to manage. It was a beautiful weekend and we rode close to 20 miles on both days. Okay, we had a fairly lengthy mid-way rest, but I felt less tired at the end of each stage than I would have done if I'd been on my own trike. The only niggle being I missed the forward view that I had on the Pino – on the trike I was looking towards Pete's back, rather than where we were going.

Wanting to be absolutely sure that we were doing the right thing, we also wanted to have a fuller trial of the Pino. We arranged to buy the second hand Pino from Kevin on the understanding that we could sell it back if it didn't prove suitable. We kept it for six weeks and rode it for a total distance of around 80 miles.

Our more extended trial revealed a serious problem that hadn't been apparent on our short initial ride. I've named this 'left knee droop'. On a recumbent your legs are stretched out, and then bent in front of you as you pedal. They need to maintain their more or less horizontal positioning. But my left leg wouldn't. After around eight miles that leg, and the knee in particular, would droop inwards. Cycling was still possible but obviously less easy, and probably wasn't doing my knee a great deal of good. So the Pino had to go back to Little Thetford and we ordered a tandem trike from George Longstaff.[1]

We took delivery of our new tandem trike in July of 2002. It has lived up to our hopes and dreams – and beyond. My view isn't just of Pete's back because I have the freedom to look around. Together we can ride further and faster. We try to ride as often as we can at the weekends. We have re-explored the Cheshire lanes which we used to ride in pre-MS days. We go out in weathers which in those days we would probably not have considered – and we enjoy it. We haven't tried to go beyond the 20 mile mark but for us that is sufficient for a good day's cycling.

Resident Mechanic and Load Mover…

Now we seem to have a fleet of cycles of one kind or another. Cycles require a degree of serious ongoing maintenance if they are to be kept on the road without major problems and breakdown at inconvenient time. I'm not really much good at this kind of thing, and I suppose I now have some excuse in that it is physically difficult for me to manage such tasks. Very fortunately for me and my continued cycling, I do have a helpful mechanic on the spot!

Having eleven wheels between us (three trikes of one kind or other plus Pete's two wheeler) means that there is plenty of opportunity to get punctures! This is a particular problem at certain times of the year. When the hedge cutters have been out the local lanes can waylay us with spiky, thorny hawthorn cuttings which slash into even supposedly puncture proof tyres. Mending punctures is certainly not Pete's favourite task but he is good at it and after a bit of cussing usually gets me or us back on the road without too much delay.

A more challenging, but more satisfying, contribution has been all the work Pete has done to improve the operation of my handcycle. For ordinary bikes there are 'rules' about how things should be set-up to achieve the comfort of the cyclist and most efficient propulsion. This is not the case in quite the same way for handcycles. Pete has put some considerable effort into achieving the best arrangement for me. He has also, importantly, improved my brakes, given me a parking brake and managed to fit mudguards to help stop me being splattered in mud. Altogether, I have got a greatly improved machine, and Pete has got satisfaction from resolving some awkward mechanical challenges.

Disabled Cycling at Home and Overseas...

As can be seen, cycling, in its various forms, has continued to be an important source of enjoyment and satisfaction for me despite the onset of disability. But what of other disabled people? Are there other disabled cyclists out there? The answer is a qualified yes. I don't think there is yet a full appreciation of the possibilities, either among disabled people themselves, or among professionals who advise on such matters. When we are out on the handcycle in particular we are frequently stopped by curious people who comment along the lines of "what a marvellous machine – we've never seen anything like it before". Among this group of interested commentators we have quite often found professional physiotherapists, or even rehabilitation specialists.

So what is going on? What source of information and provision of equipment already exists? I belong to the Handcycling Association of the UK. This was set up in 1999 and has a small but enthusiastic membership, largely of paraplegics and tetraplegics. Many members are like myself and are primarily interested in recreational cycling of one kind or another. A questionnaire investigation of the membership which I carried out showed similar pleasures and satisfactions to those which I get from my own handcycling.

There are those who achieve some quite amazing things. Members have, for example, handcycled around the whole circumference of the UK, completed a solo handcycling and camping tour around Iceland

and a party of four crossed the Karakorum Highway in the Himalayas using a recumbent tandem with hand cranking for the disabled rider. Some other members are very competitive and take part in racing and time trials, in both national and international competitions. The acceptance of handcycling as a paralympic sport has now done a great deal to increase its competitive profile.

Unfortunately, one of the major problems in relation to such equipment is the high cost[2]. These cycles cannot easily be mass produced, and there is not the kind of huge market that there is for, say, mountain bikes and so there cannot be economies of scale. Specialist bikes for disabled people are produced by small scale specialist producers. However, this does have advantages. It means that the producers are usually committed enthusiasts and adaptations for the needs of individual riders are possible.

The expense of such cycles in this country might suggest that cycling for disabled people would not be relevant to disabled people in developing countries. In actuality cycles of various kinds are used more widely, and for a greater variety of purposes, in many poorer countries. As a consequence, there are more parts available for re-use and a greater concern not to allow things to go to waste. Also cycle building is a relatively low tech operation.

Action on Disability and Development is a British based charity which works to support disabled people in 12 of the poorest countries in Africa and Asia. Their principal approach is to fund and support the setting up of self-help groups of disabled people. The argument is that in this way disabled people in these countries can be helped towards running their own lives, setting up their own organisations, and solving many of their own problems. Experience has shown that relatively small financial input can help in the setting up of small scale businesses to enable disabled people to gain greater financial independence.

However, mobility is equally an issue for disabled people in developing countries as it is over here. Photographs included in the ADD newsletter show that handcycles of one kind or another make a contribution in this respect.

It was of particular interest to read about the tricycle workshop in the town of Bobo-Dioulasso in the West African Country of Burkino Faso, which is one of the poorest of developing nations. The workshop was set up 15 years ago, and is now clearly well established, employing 20 disabled workers. The workshop is partly self-financing, but some supporting finance is provided by ADD. As well as directly providing employment, the local manufacture of handcycle tricycles enables other disabled people to gain the mobility and independence to earn their own living. Handcycles do, indeed, provide all sorts of benefits, in all sorts of places.

Notes and References

1. Very sadly George Longstaff died suddenly in October 2003. Fortunately the cycle firm which he founded, Longstaff Cycles, continues to flourish.

2. Longstaff Cycles continues to custom build single tricycles at a price of around £4,000. Their cheaper version is a modified, mass produced bike at £800, but without an electric motor. A complete tricycle with integral electric motor is, in 2009, available from Powabyke at £889.

There are a number of specialist handcycle firms in this country. Two of these are Da Vinci Mobility at www.davinciwheelchairs.co.uk and Bromakin at www.bromakin.co.uk – handcycles from these firms could be expected to cost in the region of £2,000. The best deal for a hancycle which I have seen is from Mission Cycles (at www.missioncycles.co.uk). It is called the Handy Handcycle Upright and in 2009 was advertised at £930.00.

Chapter Nine

Me and Others

Becoming disabled is an individual thing – it has happened to you and not to anybody else. In the final analysis, how you cope and manage is down to you – your responsibility. But, all of us live our lives in a social context. We are fundamentally social beings. The ways in which other people react to us, our day to day contacts with others, our friendships and close personal relationships are crucial for our well-being.

However, when you become ill and disabled these social contacts and relationships change. What has been the nature of these changes as they have happened to me? The following commentary reviews my experience, but this personal account is placed in the context of knowledge as a social psychologist.

Disclosure – Telling One's Story...

Talking to other people about what has been happening to us, and listening to what they have to tell us in return, is the basis of everyday social interaction. It also provides the basic means for getting to know somebody. We are all familiar with those conversations, perhaps at a party or other social gathering, in which we inquire of another person where they live, what their job is, whether they have children and so on. They in their turn make return inquiries. It is part of the process of beginning to get to know somebody.

Many such initial interactions will never progress any further. However, sometimes it will be the beginning of a relationship in which we gradually get to know each other better. That 'getting to know' process is likely to proceed according to certain social rules.[1] Some of these rules are to do with the way in which we disclose information to each other through ongoing interaction.

An important social rule is that as a closer relationship develops we are likely to disclose, and, in turn, receive from the other increasing personal and perhaps intimate information. This is always a finely judged business. Being on the receiving side of intimate disclosure is, in many ways, a confirming process. The other person must like and trust us, and it is likely that we will return those feelings of trust.

On the other hand, too much intimate disclosure too soon can be difficult to deal with. Anyone who makes intimate disclosures that are not reciprocated is likely to feel uncomfortably exposed. At the same time, the one who is disclosed to will probably be feeling some pressure to reciprocate at the same level of intimacy. If they do not want to do this they are also likely to experience feelings of awkwardness. So, in the early stages of a possibly developing relationship there is a complex testing and checking process involved. Proceeding gradually is usually the best strategy.

Some special occasions in which these usual 'rules of the game' are absent actually demonstrate their importance. Many of us will have experienced a situation where somebody we hardly know has disclosed to us some quite intimate parts of their life experience. Typically this can happen on a train journey. We are sitting opposite and get talking to someone, or rather they talk to us. This breaks the usual interactional conventions in that the disclosures are largely one way. However, the most important departure from a relationship situation is that when the journey ends, we will both leave the train and never see each other again. There is no risk that the potential costs of intimate disclosure will ever become actual.

Becoming disabled means that there is a somewhat different context for disclosing – or not disclosing. One of the commonest social exchanges that we all experience is when we meet up with a friend or acquaintance, to be asked: 'How are you?', 'Are you well?', 'How are things going?' We usually respond to inquiries after our welfare fairly quickly and briefly: 'Pretty well, thank you', or 'I've had a bit of a cold but it's improving now'. A familiar social interchange.

Since I've had MS, it hasn't felt quite so easy and straightforward to reply to these kinds of everyday social inquiries. I'm not really fine and quite all right. On the other hand, it is not usually the time and place to go into a longer discussion of symptoms and state of mind. My usual strategy is to answer, 'Not so bad, thank you', which covers many possibilities in a rather vague kind of way.

Of course, good friends may really want to know how you are, and a fuller discussion can follow. But it still requires rather more thought than previously to decide how much to tell in any situation. I do want some people to know what I am experiencing. On the other hand I do not want to 'go on' too much, or too long, and there are some things which I might be reluctant to disclose to any but the most trusted friends.

Some friends or acquaintances who are themselves ill, or disabled, have said to me something along the lines of, 'I can talk to you about this because you are disabled too'. I understand that reaction and I too probably will talk a bit differently in that kind of context. However, I would like to reveal something about my experiences to those of you who are not yourselves disabled. Certainly, there is no need to tell everybody I meet. But disclosure to at least some of those people who are personally important is probably psychologically beneficial. This is especially so if one then receives supportive feedback in return. I am lucky to have some friends who can offer that kind of confirmation.

Fortunately, I have a husband to whom I can talk about pretty well most things. Pete is a good listener. Maybe a rare quality in the male species, but he is ready to listen as I expand on what happens to me, and my associated feelings and reactions. Perhaps we have both got better at this kind of discussion in the period since I have had MS. Whatever, it is certainly hugely helpful to have someone close who can help in this kind of exploration.

Psychologists have researched into, and commented on, the benefits of disclosure in both written form as well as orally. One of the first psychologists to emphasise the value of disclosure was Sidney Jourard, in his 1971 book the *The Transparent Self*.[2] More recently James Pennebaker has written extensively about self-disclosure processes.[3] His research has suggested that, although there might be some pain involved, writing about traumatic events can ultimately be beneficial. He simply invited participants in his research to write about troublesome past experiences for periods of 15 to 30 minutes. These writing periods were spaced out over a number of days, either arranged consecutively, or perhaps at weekly intervals.

This is clearly not a social situation – you are not disclosing to another person. Indeed, the disclosure is wholly anonymous with the writing just being placed in a collection box at the end of the session. A possible benefit is that you do not need to worry about the interpersonal risks you might take through your disclosure. On the other hand you also miss out on the possibility of supportive reactions from another person.

Despite the degree of artificiality involved, Pennebaker found that in many ways, such disclosure appears beneficial for many respondents. For some of them there are even physiological changes such as a positive effect on immune function, and lowering of blood pressure and heart rate. There can be mood improvement and reduced medical consultations.

Pennebaker and colleagues suggest that the opportunity to work through past stressful experiences is beneficial. In support of this they have found that written disclosure accounts, in which causal words (such as because, reason), and insight words (for instance understand, realise) predicted improved health in respondents. They speculate that the disclosure experience may have helped people to make sense of past difficult or threatening experiences, enabling them to develop a more coherent and meaningful account of what has happened.

This research involved ordinary, normally healthy respondents. Those of us who are ill and disabled might well have more than our fair share of difficult life experiences to work through. Although it might not suit everybody, I have certainly felt that intermittent diary keeping helps in working things out. For me, writing this book has also contributed to this meaning making process.

How Am I Doing?

One particular form of social disclosure involves having a social, communal grumble. Although one might be grumbling about something unpleasant, difficult or unjust, having a whinge can often be a therapeutic occasion. But there must be other people with whom complaints can be shared. A satisfying grumble is a particular kind of social occasion. It requires companions who are in the same situation as oneself. Everybody has to know what it is all about and to have common cause.

When I was working, I used to get some satisfaction from a good, whinge session with colleagues. It was a way of venting frustration and making connections with others. It also contributed to the development of social and group cohesion. Thus, although a negative event might have set us off, there could be useful outcomes, both individually and in terms of group solidarity.

Now that I am not working I miss these sessions. As a disabled person, I feel that I have plenty of things to grumble about, but it is not as easy to find a fellow group of people to grumble to and with. I do, of course, know other people who are disabled, but they tend to be less easily accessible than work colleagues. It is more difficult to get a group of us together in the same situation. Also, although we might all be disabled, our experiences of disability and the problems it causes us are quite varied. It is less likely that we will have a particular, negative experience in common that can provide a common, social focus for our grumbles.

There is another reason for missing a common reference group. We gather information about how we are doing through the process of social comparison. We assess our own performance by comparison to other people with whom we come in contact. But it is better – that is more informative – if we can compare ourselves with others who are like us.

While I was teaching it was very helpful to find out about how colleagues managed various teaching situations – especially the more challenging ones. Such information could give me new ideas about how to do things, but also give me comparative information about how my own teaching was going. Complex inferential processes are unavoidable in judgements of this sort. However, such assessments become even more difficult when there isn't ready access to a comparative reference group. How can I judge how I am doing as a disabled person in the rather more isolated, in some ways more lonely, situation in which I find myself?

Comparative social information now tends to be somewhat limited. There are, however, various sources of less direct information, and I have found these alternative sources to be of considerable value. I can find out about the lives and experiences of other people with disabilities through published memoirs, TV programmes, newspaper columns, internet sites and chat rooms. There is a fair amount of information available once you start looking for it, and it is increasing. These accounts of experiences, lives and problems faced enable me to place myself within this different web of achievement. It reduces the feelings of being 'outside' and on your own.

A more obvious, but probably less frequent source of information about how one is doing comes from direct social feedback. Young children usually get plenty of encouraging comments about their success and achievement, but they tend to fade away somewhat as we get older, or at least become more ambiguous and perhaps ironic.

Giving supportive, but not over effusive, feedback in the adult context is quite a complex and subtle social skill. I am fortunate to have some friends who can and do offer such support in a way that is encouraging and helpful. I greatly appreciate this kind of direct and supportive feedback.

Sometimes such feedback can arrive quite unexpectedly. At an academic conference some years ago I got talking to a young Australian. He was able to convey his understanding of my physical limitations by telling me how restrictive he had found it recently when he had just broken his thumb. I felt that he appreciated the challenge and difficulties that I face without him having to spell things out in detail. I very much appreciated, and still treasure, his sensitive and empathic reaction.

In contrast I have met individuals who have a foot or leg in plaster and are using crutches to get about. They can see that I also am having difficulty, but without inquiring about my situation they proceed to tell me how frustrating they are finding getting about and how they can't wait to get back to 'normal'!

Getting Into Different Groups...

Becoming disabled means it is almost inevitable that the groups to which one belongs will change – to a degree at least.[4] Some of those membership changes might not be wholly welcome. At the most general you have to get used to being a member of that class of people which others label, 'the disabled'. One of the challenges is that many people who are not disabled will have negative perceptions of this overall group. Having to become a member oneself means that there is an impetus to find ways of avoiding the acceptance of these negative perceptions.

One way is to become a member of a more specific group of people with disabilities, where the group has positive aims and reasons for its existence. For me, one such important group has been the Handcycling Association of the United Kingdom. As previously explained, handcycling has become an important part of both Pete's and my recreational activity. Mostly it is something which just the two of us do. – it is a way for us to enjoy getting out into the countryside. However, it is important to know there are other people out there for whom handcycling is also significant.

Because we are a national association with a limited number of members scattered all over the country, it is not easy for members to get together. The annual general meeting, with a group ride afterwards, provides one opportunity to 'meet up'. I was a committee member for a couple of years, which provided a further opportunity to get to know at least some members more personally.

Being involved with the association has also made me appreciate the importance of newsletters as a way of encouraging feelings of belonging within a group such as this. Our newsletter is published four times a year and includes articles on routes and competition meetings, and various other bits of news. I know that I am not alone in thinking that it provides an important focus of common identity.

Another national, but much larger group of which I am a member, is the Multiple Sclerosis Society. Probably most readers will know that this is a major charity which organises research into MS, but also provides support in a whole variety of ways for people with MS.

For most of the time that I have been a member there hasn't been a great deal of personal involvement. I haven't joined the local branch of the society. This has been for a number of reasons. Especially early on, just as I was coming to terms with having MS, I felt that I didn't want to be faced with meeting a whole lot of people who were much more disabled than I was by their MS. That was more threatening than I felt I could cope with. Of course, many people with MS do face this challenge more directly than I have done, and derive considerable benefit from getting involved.

More recently I got involved in a different and more specific way. The MS Society started a Research Network of people who have MS. The purpose of setting up this group was to include people who have MS in the process of assessing applications for funding from the MS Society. Arguably, people who have MS themselves might have different – but valuable – views on which research projects should be funded.

The Network began with an initial 'teach in' meeting. This was a very positive experience for me because it involved meeting with others who were dynamic, enthusiastic and well qualified – as well as having MS. I participated in the interesting process of evaluating research applications. over a three year period. Contact with other members of the network was only by e-mail and through the network newsletter. Even so, for me, it provided a group with whom I could strongly, and positively, identify.

Stigma or Not?

Belonging to particular groups is an important part of social experience, but so is being a part of wider, broader society. Becoming disabled means that there may also be changed experiences at this level. It may be that one will meet with negative, prejudiced reactions from other members of society. At the relatively trivial level someone might show impatience when my handcycle gets in the way. More importantly and fundamentally, many people with disabilities meet with negative reactions when trying to obtain the kind of employment justified by their qualifications.

Personally, I have been fortunate. I have not experienced much in the way of negative reactions from other people. Probably, I have been protected from the worst in various kinds of ways. When I became disabled in middle age, I had already passed through that stage of establishing myself, negotiating my way through the educational system, and then obtaining employment. Most of my friends already knew about disability issues from an academic or professional perspective and so would be unlikely to have changed reactions towards me.

However, it's certainly not always like this. The charity Scope ran a publicity campaign in the autumn of 2004 to highlight examples of the prejudiced behaviour which disabled people are facing in their day to day lives. The term 'disablism' was coined as a way of labelling this. As described, my personal experience has fortunately been limited, but I still feel a strong concern over these issues.

Psychologists and sociologists have researched into, and tried to understand, the processes involved. Sociologists tend to refer to the idea of 'stigma' which describes a persistent characteristic of a person which produces negative reactions in others. They try to understand the causes of these negative reactions and their impact on the lives of those who they see as stigmatised.

The most influential sociological contribution in this area came in the work of Irving Goffman, published in 1963 as *Stigma: Notes on the Management of Spoiled Identity*. I first read his book after I had become disabled, and I found it quite a disturbing experience. His positive contribution was to emphasise that negative social responses to disability can be as great a problem as the direct limitations of the disability itself. But for me this was altogether overshadowed by the negativity, indeed the prejudice of the language he used. He refers, for example, apparently unself-consciously to 'physical deformities' and 'abominations of the body'.

He was, of course, writing quite a while ago, but I still find it surprising that he failed to appreciate the civil rights and campaigning approach in relation to disability. Similarly, he had little appreciation of the positive value of group support and solidarity within a stigmatised group. He writes, for example, that,

> *Among his own, the stigmatised individual can use his disadvantage as a basis for organising his life, but he must resign himself to a half world to do so. Here he may develop his sad tale accounting for his development of the stigma...*[5]

Psychological contributions do not underestimate the problems caused in society by prejudiced reactions. However, they have perhaps been more useful in aiding our understanding of the nature and especially the causes of these reactions. The psychological explanation of prejudice derives from investigations into the in-group and out-group feelings and attitudes to which we are all prey.

Investigations into 'minimal groups' show how readily preferences for one's own group can arise, even in quite simple situations. Tajfel and colleagues carried out the original investigation in the 1970s with Bristol schoolboys, but it has been repeated since with many different groups.[6] The boys were allocated to two groups on quite arbitrary grounds, such as their preferences for one or other of two abstract artists. But these 'groups' were not real groups. The boys knew the name of the group to which they belonged, but they never met with their fellow members. Instead, each boy was sent, by themselves, to an individual cubicle.

There, they completed a task in which they had a series of opportunities to award points, which would represent monetary reward, to two other boys, but never to themselves. The only thing they knew about the boys to whom they were awarding money was the 'abstract artist group' to which each boy belonged. Over a series of trials, boys consistently responded by awarding more money to the boy out of the pair who was described as a member of their own group. This happened even though they were not personally going to benefit. The rules of 'fair play' didn't seem to play a part.

These investigations show how easy it is to trigger preferential behaviour that has the aim of benefiting one's own group. In this research this happened in really quite artificial circumstances. The boys never met each other. They were not members of any real social group. Even so they had developed a degree of 'group loyalty' which led to prejudiced behaviour towards the other 'out group'. Real group members share histories, loyalties and badges of membership that are embedded in a complex web of social, ethnic and cultural relationships. These can, as we are all aware, reinforce further the development and maintenance of prejudice.

But why do these preferences and prejudices arise so readily? The psychological explanation of prejudice extends beyond this social and cultural reinforcement. It emphasises that our tendency to categorise the members of our social world into 'us' and 'them' is a necessary part of organising and simplifying the complexity of our social and cultural environment. Furthermore, when we start to think that 'we' are better than 'them', we soon get more personal feelings of superiority. Positive feelings of self identity derive from our membership of a successful in group, in contrast to the out group, which it is useful and beneficial for us to judge as less acceptable.

How does prejudice towards people with disabilities relate to this kind of explanatory scheme? There is a sense in which people with disabilities can constitute an 'out group' for people who are not disabled. We are different, 'them', 'the other'. There will certainly be overt, prejudiced behaviour by some who place themselves in the 'normal' grouping and identify strongly with it. For others, with stronger social consciences, it will be much more a case of awkwardness – not quite knowing the most appropriate or best way to behave.

One important difference between people who are disabled and other minority groups is that anybody might find themselves forced to join us at any time. This can have negative, but perhaps potentially more positive consequences for us, those who have disabilities. In a negative sense, it can perhaps lead to a more vehement rejection of us among those who do not wish to admit, or contemplate, that they could become disabled themselves. In this sense, we serve to highlight everyone's vulnerability to weakness, disability, pain and death – which can be threatening.

But such feelings of vulnerability also have the potential to lead to positive outcomes. Susan Wendell points out that in any reasonably prosperous society we now expect there to be facilities to treat acute or emergency health problems. Everyone is quite clear that they might need these at any time. If we had the same kind of attitude to the possibility of disability, that is 'if the non disabled saw the disabled as potentially themselves, or as their future selves', then there would be stronger motivation to ensure full accessibility and adequate financial support.[7] As Wendell emphasises, unless we die very suddenly, most people will have some experience of living with at least a degree of disability in the latter years of their lives.

Many, including quite a few psychologists, would see this as representing a rather naive optimism. Prejudiced attitudes are difficult to change because they derive from a strong cognitive pressure towards negative stereotyping of minority 'out groups'. But there is also long-standing psychological support for the argument that legislation has a role to play in changing attitudes, as well as providing legal penalties for discriminative behaviour. In spite of its limitations, the Disability Discrimination Act has provided crucial indicators that discrimination is not socially acceptable.

Well yes, but what of actual experience in the real world? As already indicated I have in many ways been fortunate in my own experience. However, I would like to comment on some of my encounters with the world which have provided a mixture of positive and negative outcomes. Admittedly, these encounters do not relate to the fundamental social areas of education and employment. But leisure and enjoyment are also an important part of life and these comments relate to the experience of getting out with my handcycle.

This machine creates considerable interest on many of our outings. Sometimes, it is just a brief passing comment, other people stop us for longer discussions. The most common reaction is along the lines of the handcycle being an amazing and wonderful machine and that they have never seen anything like it before. We quite often end up giving information about how to find out about handcycles through the internet. I think that many people are genuinely glad that it enables me to get out, as they can, to beautiful places. I am both pleased, and encouraged by their enthusiastic reactions.

A variant on the theme comes from those who contribute a degree of humour. My favourite was an occasion when we were negotiating a single track, very dusty lane. A large lorry came up behind us. There was no room for it to pass so it had to slow right down, while we carried on as quickly as we could. When we got to a suitable place we moved over to let it pass. The lorry driver rolled down his window, and commented somewhat laconically, "I couldn't see for the dust!" Humour is, it seems to me, a supportive and confirming reaction. It is an indicator that you belong to the inclusive group of ordinary humanity, and that you are not some different kind of person who has to be treated especially carefully, or is better ignored.

Other interesting reactions come from children, most particularly boys of around the ages of eight to eleven. They are enthusiastic and fascinated. "That's really wicked", or, "What a cool bike", or a shouted comment to others, "Come and see this fantastic bike". Quite often they want to know more about how it works and how fast it goes. One of the interesting things about their reactions is that they always see it as a 'bike thing' although the wheelchair origins of my handcycle are fairly evident. There doesn't seem to be any indication of awkwardness or prejudice in these reactions.

Thus, for me, these encounters are an important indication that many people out there, whom I do not know, can be friendly and supportive, and not prejudiced. But, there are other times when cycling outings can be frustrating and demonstrate that the Disability Discrimination Act certainly does not reach all important parts.

This frustration happens most often when we are out on the tandem tricycle. We do cycle on the road, but we prefer to be away from traffic when at all possible. Over recent years the Sustrans organisation has been working energetically to develop cycle routes in this country. Some of these use quiet country roads, but other parts are dedicated traffic free cycle routes, many using disused railway lines or canal paths for example. All have had considerable investment to bring them up to a good standard.

In their campaigning publicity Sustrans emphasise that their routes are not just for cyclists. They suggest that countryside access for people with disabilities is also available. However, a problem arises because they (or the local authorities who control many of the routes) are also, understandably, keen to exclude joy riding young motor bike riders. Consequently many routes include barriers designed to keep these trouble makers out. The problem is that these barriers, in their ingeniously varied forms, seem better at excluding disabled buggy riders, handcyclists and tandem tricyclists. The trail bike motor cyclists usually seem to find ways of getting through!

Partnership Dynamics...

For many people with disabilities, prejudice and discrimination need to be faced, coped with and counter-acted. But, as with everybody else, the closer, more intimate relationships and partnerships probably have a stronger and more immediate impact on our well-being.

Psychologists who study the dynamics of partnership relationships suggest that fairness, or equity within a partnership is an important quality.[8] This would probably co-incide with the interpretation which most of us make from within a partnership. We are looking for a fair relationship in which the costs and benefits are equally distributed. Ultimately, the issue of who does what, when, in relation to day to day processes of managing the minutiae of the domestic economy is important. Problems arise, of course, because of different interpretations of what is fair.

When one member of a partnership becomes disabled there are bound to be implications for both. One of the most difficult adjustments relates to changes in dependence and independence. The chronically ill and disabled partner is likely to find that they cannot do all the things that they used to. A degree of assistance needs to be given and accepted. The most obvious parallel in ordinary life comes when a couple start a family, and have a new baby. Adjustments have to be made, and a new balance achieved.

When I first developed MS in 1993, Pete and I had been married for 21 years. I think that our partnership was a generally equitable one over these years. We hadn't faced any major de-stabilising challenges. Prior to the onset of my MS we had both worked full-time with no breaks. We had developed tried and tested strategies for a fair sharing of household tasks.

So how would we cope in this new situation? After 1997, I was at home all day. I am moderately disabled so there are certainly household tasks that I can do. On the other hand, I do not have a great deal of stamina. I get tired quickly from just standing up. And I certainly wanted to do other things than just looking after the house. We have had to make new adjustments; some have been relatively easy, others more difficult.

For as long as I can remember Pete and I have shared the cooking. Frequently we cooked together, although each of us had dishes over which we felt we had prime ownership. Depending on work commitments, and what time each of us got home, one or other of us might completely prepare the meal; but more frequently there would be some degree of co-operation.

Now that I am generally at home, Pete could have expected that I would have a meal waiting for him when he arrived. Fortunately he didn't and doesn't. He accepts that I still have other things I want to do. We share the cooking in very much the way we used to, though we are perhaps now more aware of the 'cooking dynamics'.

Cooking together can sometimes provoke arguments. This mostly happens when one of us has taken over a dish that the other usually cooks. This can lead to interference and a reaction of 'Do it my way – damm you'. We usually manage to realise how silly we are being before tempers are completely lost!

The other source of aggravation to Pete is that I am a rather untidy cook, and leave things scattered around the work surface. Pete, on the other hand, has a 'tidy as you go' policy. Mind you, I can sometimes find that Pete has tidied away some piece of equipment that I haven't even finished using! But, all in all, we still very much enjoy working together in the kitchen.

Keeping control of the more general housework – the cleaning and tidying side of things has been more difficult and challenging and a source of greater tension between us. In pre-MS days it was all so simple – we took the easy way out of having somebody else do the cleaning for us. Noreen was a most excellent cleaner and got us thoroughly spick and span once a week. She worked for us from 1984 at our previous house in Alsager. When she first started, her two daughters were just at the stage of moving to secondary school. She 'came with us', as it were, when we moved to Sandbach, and continued to do her weekly clean after I had stopped working. By this time both her daughters had graduated from university.

As well as keeping us fully cleaned, Noreen had very much become a friend, and we had also got to know her husband, Cliff. Then, in 2002, Noreen got a single job that was more convenient for her than moving around for a number of cleaning jobs, and nearer to her home base on the edge of the Potteries. It was better for her, but a great loss to us. I'm pleased that the four of us have stayed friends, and we meet for a meal together on a reasonably regular basis. Clearly though, we would have to make different arrangements for keeping the house clean and tidy!

Our plan (or perhaps it should be said my plan!) was that I should do the lighter cleaning on a day to day basis. This does make me tired, but, as I've said, if I do a little bit at a time it is manageable. Pete does the hoovering when he can fit it in, which is most often on a Saturday or Sunday morning.

Pete has been keener that we should find another cleaner, which I have resisted. During the day I feel the house is very much my territory, and I am not keen to have my space invaded. I am being a bit awkward, but Noreen, as a friend, made it different. The other thing is that Pete likes to have things clean and tidy, whereas I have a greater tolerance of disorder. We have somewhat different preferences.

Another area relates to to perception over the degree of help and support that is required by the ill and disabled partner, or alternatively the continuing level of capability. It is quite possible that the two people involved could easily see the situation – and the degree of help and support that is needed – quite differently.

Psychologists have recently begun to suggest that divergent judgements and expectations about levels of disability or capability can lead to problems.[9] If the non disabled partner thinks that the other cannot do as much as they actually can, and is therefore over solicitous, and always offering assistance when that is not needed, it is likely the disabled partner will become frustrated and exasperated. On the other hand, if the able bodied partner doesn't appreciate the extent of help and support that is required, this could be just as upsetting. Quite a delicate balance is involved here.

Obviously it is advantageous if both people involved have realistic and reasonably correct perceptions. Easy to say, but not so easy to achieve. This is especially the case when levels of capability or need for support are likely to change over time, and even on a day to day basis. It is a truism to say that good levels of communication are required for any harmonious partnership, but, especially so in the context of disability and chronic illness.

The most dramatic instances of this problem for Pete and I occur when we are out exploring with the handcycle. There are occasions when Pete has somewhat inflated perceptions of where it is possible for me to go. Sometimes he can go charging off over rough, rutted, or boggy ground assuming that I will be able to follow when it isn't always realistic. On the other hand, there have been times when we get to explore interesting and rewarding paths that I might have been reluctant to investigate without his encouragement. But just sometimes I really have had to insist that discretion is the better part of valour. After all, I am the one who feels the jolts and bumps over that rocky path!

But, overall the explorations we have made by handcycle and tandem trike have been of huge benefit to us. Indeed, acquiring these machines and getting them to work in the way that we want has been an important co-operative project. Having shared challenging goals in this context has been very rewarding for both of us. All the psychological evidence suggests that working together to solve problems has a very positive pay-off in terms of encouraging good relationships and good group moral.

Okay, we are a middle aged married couple, not a newly established working group. Nevertheless, the positive feelings that come from the joint project of achieving better mobility for me, and finding better ways of getting out to beautiful places together, provide a great sense of success and emotional satisfaction. Despite the challenges (or maybe because of them) we are still finding that wheeling through life together is working for us.

But, inevitably, living in partnership after the onset of disability doesn't work for everybody. The level of adjustment and re-adjustment required can be too high. Divorce rates do increase in these circumstances. In some cases it can be the disabled partner who takes the initiative. Early on I read of one lady who had not been altogether happy in her marriage. When she developed MS she decided that she couldn't tolerate both MS and an unsatisfactory husband. Since it was impossible to get rid of the MS, she decided that she needed to ditch the husband, a hugely courageous decision.

Since reading that account I have got to know Mary, who made a similarly difficult and courageous decision. The story starts with my earlier meeting with Martin, another Sandbach resident who has MS. We met out on the street. I was riding my trike and Martin was on his electric scooter. We started talking, which led on to us becoming friends. Martin had developed MS in his mid thirties and it put paid to his career as a musician and music teacher. He had earlier had an organ scholarship at one of the Oxford colleges.

When I met Martin in 2000 he was living independently in a bungalow in the grounds of Sandbach Leonard Cheshire home. He was coping well and had made other friends in and around Sandbach. He was well known in the town as he drove his electric scooter around its streets quite fast. But I knew that he was a bit lonely.

Then Mary, who also has MS, left her husband in Alsager, and moved into another of the Leonard Cheshire bungalows. They became friends, and it progressed from there. Soon they had moved together into an attractive little cottage nearer the centre of Sandbach, but in a nice secluded spot. Pete and I were really delighted to be able to join in the celebration of their marriage in the summer of 2006. It was a very special day.

Inevitably it has not been altogether easy for them. They both have MS. Martin's condition deteriorated, necessitating full time wheelchair use. Mary's MS has a relapse-remission form, so coping abilities are pushed hard when a relapse occurs. The occasional difficult times are worked through with great determination. When we see them they are usually remarkably positive and cheerful. Now they are both our friends. Mary is a very warm, friendly and resourceful person. Music is still very important in Martin's life although he is no longer able to play the organ. He is still regularly out and about on the streets of Sandbach, and his sense of humour is definitely intact. I very much admire the way that they have coped with the various challenges which they have faced in their life together.

Difference and 'Otherness'…

The discussion in this chapter has been about maintaining relationships with other people. But inevitably the onset of illness and disability means that this has been in a changed context. I think that I have been lucky to escape some of the experiences of prejudice and discrimination which others experience. At the same time I do not think that anyone who enters into this new world can wholly escape a sense of being different.

This sense of difference has been brought home to me recently. This was through an experience which involved sadness and loss. But it was also an experience which emphasised the value of discussing and working through difficult experiences with other people. After a long, and fulfilling life my father died at the beginning of 2005. It wasn't altogether a shock – he had been ill with cancer for a few months, though the end, as a result of pneumonia, was still unexpected.

But this was something that I could share with other people, knowing that many of my friends had already been through this experience. The death of any parent is a life-stage event which we all have to negotiate our way through – so we can share things, discuss reactions and compare them with those of others, whilst sorting out our own feelings.

Such sharing and support are less available when one becomes ill and disabled. There are other people who will offer sympathy and concern. But they cannot, however sympathetic they are, discuss on the basis of common experience. Of course, there are many people in the world out there who will have been through similar experiences, and finding out how it has been for them and how they have managed is useful. But it is not quite the same as having friends around you, the friends you have always had, who have been through things with you, and can talk with you on the basis of shared life events.

This absence contributes to the sense of difference, and 'otherness', that comes with disability. It is part of what is happening. It cannot be ignored. So how do I react and cope? One reaction, which has emerged strongly since the time when Goffman was writing about stigma in relation to disability, is the pride which minority group members take in their own identity. However, I'm not convinced that being proud to *be* disabled is a fully justified reaction. *Being* disabled is something that just happens to one, but we who are disabled should certainly take pride in *coping* with disability, an achievement that needs to be celebrated.

There is another way in which this sense of difference can contribute to positive outcome. Susan Wendell emphasises that 'otherness' derives from cultural and social experience and pressures, but it can limit that experience. Not being able to easily talk about one's experience of disability is personally limiting, but Wendell suggests it is also limiting to those who are not disabled:

...it deprives the non-disabled of the knowledge and perspectives that people with disabilities could contribute to culture, including knowledge of how to live well with physical and mental limitations.[10]

We have not yet reached that ideal level of easy integration and there are probably reasons why it might never be possible.

Currently, those of us who are ill and disabled have to straddle both worlds – and such straddling is not always the most comfortable position. Nevertheless, with moderate optimism (or maybe just naivety), I believe most of us in the world of disability are struggling to bridge the two, seeking to bring some of the non-disabled with us, rather than resigning ourselves to the stigmatised half world that Goffman identified. We can seek to use the sense of 'otherness' in a way which extends cultural experience as Wendell suggests would be advantageous. We can also use the sense of difference and 'otherness' to support our sense of personal identity and positive achievement.

Notes and References

1. There is considerable psychological literature which examines this process of getting to know someone as mediated through self-disclosure. A useful overview is provided in Derlega, V. J., Metts, S., Petronio, S. & Margulis, S. T. (1993). *Self-Disclosure*. Newbury Park, Ca: Sage Publications.

2. Jourard, S. M. (1971). *The Transparent Self* (2nd ed.). New York: Van Nostrand Reinhold.

3. Pennebaker has carried out extensive research into disclosure in the context of coping with health related difficulties and threats. One overview publication is Pennebaker, J. W. (1997). *Opening Up: The healing power of expressing emotion.* (2nd Ed.). New York: Guilford.

4. The whole area of group membership and experiences of personal and group identity within the groups to which one belongs is an important one within social psychology. A textbook which provides an introduction to some of the ideas which are used within this section is Hogg, M.A. & Abrams, D. (1988). *Social Identifications*. London: Routledge.

5. Goffman, E. (1963). *Stigma: Notes on the management of a spoiled identity*. New York: Simon and Schuster. p.20. There is a good critical account of Goffman's work in chapter 3 of *The Rejected Body* by Susan Wendell which was referred to previously.

6. Tajfel, H. (1981). *Human Groups and Social Categories*. Cambridge: Cambridge University Press provides a discussion of this and later research.

7. The quotation is from Wendell, S. (1996). *The Rejected Body*. New York: Routledge. p.53.

8. A recent article which investigates relationship equity in the context of illness and disability is Kuijer, R. G., Buunk, B. P. & J. F. Ybema. (2001). Intimate relationships when one partner of a couple has cancer. *Social Psychology Quarterly*, 64, 3, 267-282.

9. One of these contributions is Morrison, V. (2001). The need to explore discrepant illness cognitions when predicting patient outcome. *Health Psychology Update*, 10 (2), 9-13.

10. Susan Wendell provides a good discussion of issues of 'otherness' in relation to disability in her book *The Rejected Body* (New York: Routledge). The quotation is from p. 65.

Chapter Ten

Models, Moods and Mindfulness

Models and Heroes...

Having and admiring heroes is, perhaps, a somewhat adolescent preoccupation. It is seen as something that people grow out of. Do you need heroes and models in middle age? I think that *I* do. These heroes, these other people, unknown to them, have a role in helping me to maintain a positive frame of mind.

Like many others, when I first became chronically ill and disabled, I had no direct experience of what was going to be involved, for it was a whole new and unknown world. As someone who was now disabled, I needed to get to know how to live with and manage that disability at a practical, but also emotional level.

I read the books about coping with and managing MS, and these were important and useful, but I also wanted something else, something more direct, and more personally engaged. It was soon evident that there are people who have written about what it is like to become ill and disabled. From early on after my MS diagnosis, I kept a look out for relevant autobiographical accounts, and now have quite a collection of book length published autobiographies of people who have faced and coped with a whole variety of disabling conditions.

So, what have I learned from other people's lives? How have I benefited from reading these various accounts? At the most general level I think it is a matter of inspiration. In this sense they really are heroes and heroines, as far as I am concerned. Their accounts help me to say to myself that if they can survive, manage, and make a positive life for themselves – then so can I!

Of course, the writers of these autobiographies come in all shapes and sizes. Disabled people are certainly not a homogeneous group. Just like other members of the human race, they come from different backgrounds, have different personal qualities, attitudes, capabilities, goals etc. So, as models they are certainly not for slavish imitation. It is more a case of picking out, identifying, particular aspects of another's responses to disability, which resonate with one's own life and style of adaptation. I have already in this book made passing comment on some such examples.

There are many others whom I could mention, but I restrict myself to a choice of two individuals who provide what, at first, might seem somewhat unlikely personal inspiration. They are both male. Both are mountaineers. Both, in quite different ways, have encountered serious incapacity – but incapacity which is quite different from my own.

One of the most amazing autobiographies I have come across is that of Erik Weihenmayer.[1] His disability made itself fully evident in middle adolescence – although his sight was quite severely limited from infancy. Initially this American teenager's reaction to going blind was rebellious non-adaptation.

The turning point probably came when he went on a summer camp which encouraged trying out various sports and outdoor activities. One of these was rock climbing – not the most obvious sport for blind teenagers. But, after feeling his way successfully up a rock face or two, Eric was beginning to become captivated by this climbing business.

I was overwhelmed by the sensation of the mountain, by the wind at my back, by the brilliant textures of the rock, the intermittent patterns of coolness and heat under my touch. It was as though my senses had awakened. Every sound, smell and touch was so vivid, so brilliant, it was almost painful.

Soon afterwards, he persuaded his father and brothers into a hike along the narrow, precipitous paths of the Inca Trail in Peru. But this was just the beginning. After more summer treks in mountain country, and then gradually more demanding ascents, Weihenmayer was excelling in the kind of physical activity in which one would never expect a blind person to become involved. He is now a serious mountaineer – who has climbed some of the highest and most challenging peaks, culminating in the ultimate mountaineering challenge – Everest.

My second hero is Jamie Andrew.[2] He became disabled as a consequence of a mountaineering adventure that went seriously wrong. In January 1999, Jamie and his climbing partner were making an attempt on a 4,000 metre Alpine Peak. They had set off from Chamonix in good weather, but then became caught high up on the mountain in a storm that went on for five days.

By the time Jamie Andrew was rescued by helicopter his partner was dead and he was suffering from hypothermia and severe frostbite. In spite of efforts by doctors, his frost-bitten hands and lower legs could not be saved and had to be amputated. So, drastically and shockingly he had become a quadruple amputee.

Three months after his near death above Chamonix, Jamie was taking his first steps on artificial lower legs. After some trials with prosthetic arms he made a different kind of adjustment. He now largely manages using his above wrist stumps. His descriptions of how he got to master various everyday tasks make a strong impression. But the most amazing story within his autobiography is that of how, despite everything, he has been able to get back to climbing mountains.

The achievements of Jamie Andrews and Erik Weihenmayer are, by any standards, remarkable and outstanding. But what do they mean for me, and to me? I don't, and never have had, any ambition to do serious mountain climbing. There isn't any kind of 'fix' that is going to make it possible for me to venture up even much lower mountains – or hills. I am inspired, but that inspiration isn't going to translate into any kind of action – so is it of any value?

The answer is yes, for me there is a value, not so much in the achievements themselves, for these cannot be emulated. Rather, the value comes in identifying, and appreciating in detail, the qualities, skills and capabilities that have made these achievements possible. Qualities such as determination, persistence, risk taking and optimism, play an essential part in coping with disability, even at much more mundane levels. Both of these mountaineers have a very strong problem facing orientation. They tackle them head on and make sure that they find solutions. Each of them finds satisfaction and enjoyment in meeting these challenges.

Jamie Andrew commented early in his recovery period that "There was no way I'd gone through hell on that mountain to come down and be miserable. So I decided to be happy". There may be some queries about whether one can 'decide' to be happy, but this comment is both salutary and thought provoking.

Not all people with disabilities would share my approval. Some might designate Weihenmayer and Andrews as belonging to the 'supercrip' category. This is not intended as a complementary term, although it is perhaps as much to do with media representation as with the individuals themselves.

If understood correctly, two main points are being made. Firstly, it is suggested that if an ordinary person sees some disabled people achieving so much, then they might think that any and every disabled person ought to be able to do the same. Secondly, it is argued that these outstanding achievements have been supported and made possible by exceptional resources. Such a level of support could then detract from what is available for other more ordinary disabled people. I have certainly heard this position being taken in relation to paralympic athletes.

This is not a position I can accept. We should celebrate and applaud the exceptional achievements of disabled people, as we do with the similar achievements of non-disabled individuals. Of course, we need to continue our campaigns for appropriate support, resources and arrangements for accessibility. These are essential, but so is the recognition of outstanding success in physical achievement, and in other fields. The success of the Paralympics demonstrates the extent to which both disabled and non-disabled spectators can enjoy performance in this context.

A Mood Review...

There will always be some days better than others. On some days things just generally go well. The coffee at breakfast tastes just right; the journey to work is without hold-ups; the boss pays us a compliment – and so on. Sometimes it is difficult to know whether we just got out of bed 'on the right side', or whether the pleasant things that have happened put us into a good mood. Other days, things can be just the reverse. Nothing goes right, and we feel generally disgruntled with the world, and find it difficult to climb out of the consequential negative mood.

Experiencing different moods is part of life. Until recently, moods (as against more long term personality differences, and more transient emotions) have been somewhat neglected by psychologists. But that is beginning to change and there have been recent useful reviews of the nature and experience of moods.[3]

But what *are* moods exactly? One useful way to try to understand the nature and experience of moods is to make a comparison with emotions. Moods tend to be longer lasting than emotions, certainly lasting hours, and maybe days. Moods usually do not have a clear cut start and finish. They can emerge somewhat mysteriously, but perhaps out of a combination of minor, hardly noticed events. Moods are weaker and less intense than emotions, but are sometimes more persistent and nagging. Moods are often unfocused evaluative states, which are not about anything in particular, but they can still have a powerful influence on our ongoing sense of well-being – or otherwise.

How can we describe the content, or feeling tone of our moods? It is probably the case that descriptions of mood characteristics offered in the literary context are more detailed, subtle and sophisticated than those offered by psychologists. The latter emphasise the importance of just two main dimensions. One of these extends from moods that are positive and pleasant at one end, to negative and unpleasant at the other. The second dimension relates to the degree of activation or arousal. Thus an annoyed mood would have a moderate level of both activation and negative tone; boredom would be negative, but with a much lower degree of activation; a euphoric mood would be positive and aroused; while a mood of calm contentment would be positive and pleasant, but with a lower level of activation.

How do we react to our own moods? Most of us would surely say that we prefer to be in a positive, pleasant mood. There are both empirical and subjective indicators that we may well make an effort to get ourselves out of a negative mood. Subjectively, we know that this sometimes works, but on other occasions is less successful, and we seem to be 'stuck' in that ongoing sense of lowness.

It is likely that some individuals are better than others at this management of their moods. It is probable that this capacity is linked to the number and variety of mood change strategies that we are able to use. Psychologists beginning to investigate the procedures which people make use of to change their moods have identified two hundred such strategies.[4]

None of us are likely to be aware of all of these, but probably most of us have developed our own personal set of 'mood changers' over the years which work for us. Common approaches are to have a set of slightly indulgent treats to which we have ready access, and to know ways in which we can relax and 'turn off' the stresses of the moment. Having someone who we know will listen to our grumbles, and who is likely to be able to cheer us up, is also helpful. It could be useful though, in good and positive times, to make some effort to extend that list.

It will come as no surprise to readers that a very important 'mood busting' strategy for me comes from getting out and about and taking exercise. My most dependable way of improving my mood is to get out on my handcycle, or tricycle. The improved mood derives from being active, having a change of scenery, and getting to pleasant places. Also, I know that I am lucky, privileged even, that I can get out in this way.

There are, of course, times when I feel frustrated at the limitations in my life. I can get somewhat 'down' as a consequence. But these feelings of privilege remind me that there are others worse off. Psychologists refer to the process of 'downward comparison'. In some ways it can feel that I am taking advantage of those who are worse off than I am.

But, it is better for my well-being (and that of other people) to make at least some such downward comparisons. It is too easy in our modern world to find ourselves pushed into upward comparisons with those who are better, or better off, than we are. There are exciting and inviting images all around us, but we all know that envy does not provide a good basis for positive mood.

It can be difficult but careful selection of comparison others has major benefits. I think that the experience of being chronically ill and disabled has encouraged me to be more careful about the comparisons I make. The major advantage of mental comparison is that we are free to compare ourselves with whomever we want to, and we can make as many comparisons as we wish, and beyond the present time. I find that making use of historical and international comparisons can be a salutary process. Here, the objective is not to feel that one is better than others, but to show how fortunate one is – which provides a good antidote to feeling incapable, and sorry for oneself.

Management strategies do not necessarily involve getting out of that negative mood. If I know from past experience that the mood is likely to improve within a reasonable period of time, then there can be advantages in accepting and tolerating it for the present. It can be an appropriate strategy for those of us who are chronically ill and disabled. We do, after all, have good reason to be sad and melancholic on occasion. I don't enjoy feeling melancholic. On the other hand, if I tell myself that accepting it for the time being seems the best thing to do, it doesn't seem so bad. In this way, acceptance of short term negative mood can, provide a positive way of dealing with that mood.

There are occasions, though, when I realise that I have a greater ability to modify my mood than I am often prepared to admit. This most obviously happens when I feel miserable and upset – but then unexpected visitors arrive. A certain degree of positive self-presentation is required. I don't want to publicly display my unhappy mood. At first a certain degree of almost artificial effort is required. But then you find that the mood really has lifted and changed.

Persistence of low mood is really a key matter here. As was previously mentioned negative mood can 'tip over' into more sustained depression that might necessitate some stronger action. So, what has been my experience in relation to ongoing mood states? What has been the nature of my 'mood history' since I developed MS in 1993.

As I have commented in other parts of this book, there have, inevitably, been 'ups' and 'downs'. There was certainly an initial period of grieving for the things that I had lost and in relation to the changes in my life that I was forced to make. However, I was then lucky because things did improve quite quickly and quite markedly.

The second relapse was, in some ways, more difficult and more upsetting because things didn't improve. Becoming reconciled to this lack of improvement was not easy. I think, though, that I did see this very much as a challenge. Also, there were interesting and important things going on in my life. I was enjoying working on my PhD, and both Pete and I were very much involved in the excitement of the build of our new house.

But then, over the period from the end of 2002 to the late Spring of 2003, things became more difficult. This was not as a direct result of changes in my MS. At that time (and this continues) the MS was largely stable. It could have been that I was finally recognising that there was no hope of improvement and that this made a contribution to the down turn in my mood.

It was also at this time that I began to think ahead to the future rather more, and perhaps became rather too focused on that. I had realised for some time that I would not be able to have the kind of active retirement I had once anticipated. But now, as I was really leaving the academic world, these two losses loomed over my life.

Alongside this, my pre-occupation was considering where we should live after Pete retired. I love our present house, and I like Sandbach and its surroundings. But as we get older, and especially if anything happened to Pete, and I was on my own, I wondered if it would be the best place for me.

In such a situation there would be many attractions to moving back to my original home town of Aberystwyth. The problem is that although the main town centre is reasonably flat, much of the housing away from the centre is not. Finding a suitable house to live in as a disabled person would not be easy. There didn't seem to be a solution, but there were times when I became pre-occupied with the mental search. Such unproductive worrying was not helpful to my mood.

Fortunately, as the Spring came these pre-occupations gradually eased. I managed to escape from these negative thoughts. At this time of year enjoyable holidays can help to support better cheer. My ongoing attempts to improve my mood with various psychological strategies were also, I think, having some impact. But this period of low spirits made me realise how easy it would be to become properly depressed.

Being Depressed…

We do use the word depressed to refer to a *mood* of being rather 'down', negative and somewhat miserable. We say 'I'm feeling a bit depressed'. But a full scale clinical depression is rather different from this and more serious. It is more sustained and persistent, and more encompassing.

Depression is clearly a concern for people with MS and other chronic diseases and disabilities. There are almost certainly more frustrations in our lives that can easily get us into a negative mood. But we also face the kind of extended life-experiences which can easily push that poor mood into longer term depression. Chronic illness can mean the continued experience of unpleasant physical symptoms. Then there is the loss of taken for granted physical capability and mobility, and perhaps the loss of previous, much enjoyed leisure activities…and so it goes on.

Paul Gilbert is one of the psychologists who has written extensively about the nature and experience of depression.[5] So, what does a more serious depression feel like? Gilbert summarises by suggesting that important changes are likely in the person's experience of motivation, emotions, thinking, social behaviour and images of life.

In motivational terms Gilbert says that we are likely to feel apathetic, have little interest, and everything seems pointless. The dominant emotional response is probably lack of capacity for pleasure and enjoyment, but there might also be anger and irritability. Depression can also affect our ability to concentrate and settle to things, and our memory. In turn, these changes influence our social relationships. Partners and friends might not understand what has happened to us, and conflicts can develop. If these kinds of responses occur within a persistent depression, it is hardly surprising if our image of life becomes a rather black and gloomy one. The world has become a different kind of place, and our lives have changed.

So, how many of us are susceptible? The quick answer is quite a lot. It is relatively common in the general population. Gilbert states that the lifetime risk for an episode of serious depression can be as high as around one in four or five, The lifetime percentage risk for men is 5% to 12%, but for women it is 10% to 26%. This may be a reflection of different ways in which men and women tend to deal with stress with men being more likely to project anger outwards.

But what are the particular conditions and events which can lead any of us into some experience of ongoing depression rather than a more transient low mood? Of course these are complex and will vary between individuals. They will include genetic susceptibility, but also, most likely, some precipitating environmental conditions. These might include such stresses as losing one's job, relationship problems and marital separation, financial problems, and so on. Becoming chronically ill and disabled is certainly one of these potential stressors, and has the added pressure that, for many of us, such a condition is likely to be permanent.

There is evidence that people who have a chronic illness, and/or a disability have an increased susceptibility to depression. The patterns of incidence differ somewhat, depending on the nature of the illness or disability. In MS for example there is evidence that around 50% of people with the disease are likely to experience one or more episodes of depression at some time in their lives, which contrasts with perhaps up to around 20% in the general population.[6] There is no clear evidence as yet that greater incidence of depression is associated with having had the disease for a longer period of time, or with greater severity.

It therefore seems likely that having MS makes one more susceptible to depression than one would have been without it. Probably this is also true for other chronic illnesses. At the same time, it is important to emphasise that most of us are not depressed most of the time. So, is there anything that we can do?

Treatment, or Prevention?

Depression can be a serious problem for many people, both those with and without serious health problems and disabilities. Psychiatrists, psychologists, and also drug companies, have given considerable attention to researching into treatment possibilities. There are two main categories of approach. These are, firstly, drug treatments and, secondly, psychotherapy of one kind or another. These two are certainly not in opposition to each other. For many people they are best used in a complementary way. For anybody who is becoming seriously depressed the starting point for identifying the most appropriate treatment plan has to be a GP consultation.

The concern here is with depression that is not so serious – a somewhat low mood that seems to be going on a bit longer than usual, or longer than you would wish. (Although, of course, what counts as a serious, or not so serious, depression, can be difficult to judge.) The suggestion is that in these less severe cases a preventative approach may be of value. Indeed, there are probably good reasons for anyone who has any susceptibility to low mood to give some thought to prevention.

So, how might prevention work? Probably the most widely used therapy approach used in relation to depression is Cognitive

Behaviour Therapy (CBT). There is considerable research evidence to support its success as a treatment method and some of its principles and strategies can be adopted for 'self help' use.

Over recent years, a number of books have been published which explain the basic rationale for CBT for the general reader. One of the best of these is 'Managing Your Mind', written by two clinical psychologists. Gillian Butler and Tony Hope.[7] Their analogy is with keeping fit as a preventative approach in relation to physical health. In the same way they argue that 'mental fitness' can help us manage our personal, emotional lives, and relationships with greater effectiveness.

The central assumption underlying CBT is that cognitive reactions to our ongoing experiences lead to emotional responses. All of us think about, and reflect on, our ongoing experience and behaviour. We 'talk to ourselves' about what is going on. Often we are hardly aware that we are doing it – it becomes largely automatic. One kind of automatic thought is when we react to many events and experiences in a negative kind of way – 'I can't do that', 'What a dreadful day' 'I can't walk properly anymore – I feel like I can't do anything!'. Of course pretty well everybody, disabled or not, has such negative reactions on occasion. But if these negative judgements and emotions become dominant, a habitual way of reacting to our lives, then this can easily contribute to sliding into a depressed state of mind.

An important objective of CBT, in the context of depression, is to help people to change these negative thoughts and assumptions – to show how and why they cannot be correct, and to encourage different and more positive judgements. If the negative judgements are well entrenched and range quite widely in the person's life then it is likely that therapy will be required to achieve change. CBT is quite a focused and direct approach to therapy. In a supportive context it enables people to experiment a bit with how they react to, and judge their own behaviour, and make changes in this. A therapist can help to show how some of the beliefs held, and judgements made just cannot be true, and encourage the client to substitute more positive, appropriate and adaptive ones.

People who are not really depressed, but perhaps feel that they are on the verge, or at risk of becoming so, are perhaps in a better position to take some action to help themselves. This is not the place to fully explore the possibilities. As indicated, there are other books which are able to do this in more detail. However, it is perhaps worth exploring a few aspects which, as a person with disabilities, I have found of value in my attempts to avoid being pulled into depression.

There are three of these on which I want to comment, but they are all inter-related to each other. Depression is to do with a loss of pleasure and enjoyment in life. Those of us who are disabled are probably more susceptible, because at least some of the things that used to give us pleasure are now lost. Consequently, we need to make a more deliberate, and determined effort to cultivate positive life experience.

So, my first suggestion is that it is worth trying to really celebrate positive achievements. We may have been conditioned into public modesty but there is no need, or reason to be so in the privacy of one's own personal evaluations. We should savour and enjoy our successes – both large and small – for all that they are worth. It may seem artificial and just too deliberate, but it is possible to cultivate the habit of doing this with a degree of subtlety.

Secondly, it can be advantageous to deliberately recognise that being disabled does pose very real challenges and difficulties. We cannot really avoid that recognition; it is an essential part of our lives, but there are different ways of making it. The problems and difficulties that accompany disability can be variously annoying, frustrating, upsetting. Nevertheless, they also provide an opportunity to 'get in' an extra sense of achievement. Coping positively with these frustrations justifies a private 'pat on the back'. More than that, it should be an important contribution to feelings of self-worth. We should feel altogether pleased with how well we are doing in difficult circumstances.

Another more wide-ranging approach to noting one's achievements often recommended within CBT, and which I have certainly found useful, is that of keeping some kind of diary. One can quite easily think at the end of the day, especially if one is not in employment, 'What on earth have I done with the day?' The day seems to have just disappeared to no effect. I have found that keeping some kind of record can be a useful way of identifying achievements. A variant on this is to require oneself to record at the end of the day (say) four positive, enjoyable happenings. Even if these are apparently small and insignificant, bringing them to attention can be beneficial.

But what kind of achievements are worth celebrating? It is all too easy to set goals and standards which are too demanding. Then there is never much chance to celebrate success. It is valuable to learn to celebrate the small things, to enjoy experiences for their own sake, and to a degree to be 'easy on oneself'. I have had to make a real effort, which is certainly not always successful, to take pleasure in doing things SLOWLY. But I think that I am getting there!

Some of these suggestions might seem too simple and banal. They might also appear as just common sense – things that most of us might do anyway. But work on depression suggests that this is not always the case. When our mood is low and negative, we can forget, or fail to use, these sensible strategies. Also, when we become disabled our usual standard setting strategies can come under stress. It is more difficult to find things to celebrate. Therefore, a deliberate, planned effort to make appropriate changes can pay dividends. With experience and practice, they become an accepted and almost taken for granted part of how you operate and manage your life.

Self Awareness and Mindfulness...

The strategies for managing mood and depression discussed above require a degree of self awareness; it is necessary for us to pay attention to our own cognitive processes – the thoughts that we have about ourselves and our behaviour. To what extent is this kind of response useful and helpful to us – or could it instead be counterproductive? The traditional recommendation that it is beneficial to 'Know Thy Self' summarises one possibility.

An alternative view is that too much self-focused attention can have negative consequences. Psychologists have researched into such self-focused awareness by requiring the completion of challenging tasks when a mirror is positioned nearby.[8] In such a situation respondents are, indeed, likely to have a heightened awareness of not reaching expected standards.

Many of us would probably agree, on the basis of our own experience, that self preoccupation can easily become negative in character. Psychologists refer to negative and repetitive ruminative thoughts – obsessive worrying about a problem from which we cannot escape. We may feel that we are tackling the problem so we keep worrying. But in our negative frame of mind such thoughts can easily lead to spiralling dejection and provide a basis for more serious depression.

However, reflective self awareness, can also be more positive. Some of the strategies of cognitive behaviour therapy just described can contribute here. Also, Bandura's ideas about self regulation, referred to previously, are valuable.[9] In those earlier comments the latter two stages of his three part model were emphasised. These were self-judgement processes – our assessment of how well we are doing in relation to our own personal standards, and to social norms; and secondly, self-reaction processes, through which we reward ourselves when we reach these standards – and so motivate ourselves towards the achievement of future goals.

But in Bandura's model the first stage of self-regulation is necessarily, and logically, self-observation, or self awareness. If we wish to have some influence over our own reactions and behaviour, then we must first of all be aware of what is going on. We must attend to, and notice our own responses.

These three sets of processes, when used appropriately, provide the means through which we can manage and regulate our own behaviour. The effectiveness with which we do this will vary depending on the adequacy of our self observation, the standards we adopt and the judgements we make of our performance and the extent to which we reward ourselves for our achievements. Ideally, Bandura suggests that an effective self-regulatory system is able to provide us with a continuing source of motivation and personal satisfaction.

When these processes are working well they support positive management of our lives, and can help to avoid depression. Of course, it isn't always that easy, especially in the context of lives changed by the advent of disability. So, how could this work in practice? The challenge of maintaining exercise after the onset of disability provides an experience of the three stages in operation. In my own case I have had these in mind as I have taken my regular walks down 'my' lane.

I try to be aware of and notice how I am walking. How is my balance? To what extent do I need to be using my sticks? When do feelings of tiredness begin to impinge? Sometimes I try to see if I can walk a bit faster, or walk a little further. At the same time I try not to be discouraged if this is not possible. I am pleased that I can walk. I can look back and know that I am walking a little better than I was a few years ago. I am pleased with myself for having made the effort to keep walking.

A rather different interest in awareness derives from the literature on meditation, deriving from its Buddhist roots. As I have mentioned, although I am by no means an experienced meditator, I have made some investigation here and I do try to meditate as regularly as I can. So, how is awareness conceived of in this context? Are there any links, or is there a contrast with self-awareness in the context of self management, as discussed above?

Awareness or mindfulness is an important goal of meditative practice.[10] Mindfulness involves focusing with clarity and precision upon what is occupying the mind at the moment. Mindfulness is achieved through the practice of concentration on some immediate focus. Traditionally, the concentration and focus is on counting the breath and its in and out movement. When thoughts or emotions disrupt this concentration, these should be gently, but firmly dismissed in order to return to the present focus on the breath. That experience of dismissal is an important one.

This would appear to involve a rather different kind of awareness to that which is involved in the self-regulation process. That, necessarily involves analysis, evaluation and judgements in relation to ongoing thoughts, experiences and responses. On the other hand, meditation involves cultivating a non-judging attitude to what comes up in the mind.

Meditation is not just a sitting activity. One can meditate while walking. This is not walking to get somewhere but walking to concentrate on the walking. One tries to be aware of taking each step – the lifting and putting down of each foot and the associated shifts in balance. Again it is focus and concentration which is of the essence.

But what about 'real life' and everyday activities? The meditative life also requires that mindfulness is practised more generally. Such daily life mindfulness involves a focus on the 'here and now', the present moment, in whatever we are doing. As a person with disabilities, I feel that this is a valuable emphasis. I know that it is all too easy to get embroiled in and worried about the future, and to lose concentration on and enjoyment of the present. Attempting to take a mindful stance to all sorts of daily tasks and experiences – from doing the dishes, to taking a shower or eating a meal – can be a valuable antidote. But, as with sitting and walking meditation, purpose and effort is required.

In some ways, cognitive behaviour therapy and self-regulation processes can seem in conflict with each other, but there can perhaps also be useful interaction. At other times they can provide useful alternative perspectives on experience. My walk down the lane can be examined, as previously, in self-regulatory terms. It can also be viewed and enjoyed as a walking meditation in which I concentrate on the feeling and pleasure of my steps, and my perceptions of the natural world around.

I have been interested and excited recently to find that important links have been made between cognitive behaviour therapy and mindfulness meditation. This has led to a new therapy approach named Mindfulness Based Cognitive Therapy.[11] This approach was developed by a small group of researchers who were focusing on depression. Their major goal was to try to find ways of reducing relapse in people who had experienced past episodes of serious depression. They found evidence that introducing such individuals to meditation and mindfulness over a series of experiential sessions provided benefits for coping more effectively with any further depressive episodes. A more recent book *The Mindful Way through Depression* is addressed directly to the individual who is experiencing depression.[12]

Happiness or Not?

Is trying to be happy anything more than seeking to avoid low mood and feelings of depression? Jamie Andrews wrote that he had decided to be happy. Can one so decide?

Over the years a number of psychologists have written about happiness, and the possibility of its achievement. Two recent contributions are by Martin Seligman, who writes about *Authentic Happiness*, and Daniel Nettle, whose book is just entitled, *Happiness*.[13] Both have some interesting and useful things to say. Over recent years the promotion of happiness has been receiving more popular attention with television programmes and even politicians getting involved.

In the past, levels of happiness were mostly taken pretty much for granted – not that I was happy all the time, but if I had been asked whether I was happy, I would have said that generally, yes, I was.

But what is happiness? It is a concept about which philosophers have long argued, with psychologists making a more recent entry to the discussion. Nettle's proposal of a three-way, or three-level model provides a useful contribution. The kind of judgement offered above represents an overall weighing up and balancing of the good and not so good parts of one's life. In Nettle's model, this is level two happiness – a cognitive judgement about where one stands in the happiness stakes.

So what about the other two levels? Level one happiness represents immediate feelings of joy or pleasure. It is an emotional feeling rather than any kind of cognitive weighing up. Often it happens unexpectedly, say, from suddenly meeting an old friend, or achieving an important goal that was by no means guaranteed. As we all know, it is joyous, can be overwhelming, but also more calmly pleasurable. It is an important part of the good life. The limitation of this kind of happiness is that it is short lived and relatively transitory. We get used to it quickly and it fades away – the celebration is over. But joyous events can be cultivated and arranged in a skilled way.

Level three happiness is perhaps less closely related to our common sense understanding of the concept of happiness. It involves a rather broader fulfilment of potential, feelings of personal growth, autonomy and self-directedness. There may be greater requirements for self understanding. There has to be some conscious appreciation of the potential goals being sought, though there may be a struggle to reach that potential. But, if we are lucky, such struggle can give rise to important and sustained feelings of inner joy and achievement. The experience of 'flow', discussed earlier, is linked to this kind of happiness.

So, am I happy now – now that I have got MS? It has become more difficult to say. I tend to think, if that is not a contradiction in terms, that achieving happiness now demands more hard work, more effort.

One of the constraints for everybody, for which there is now quite strong psychological evidence, is that happiness is influenced to a fair degree by inheritance. Some people are temperamentally more cheerful, bubbly, happy-go-lucky than others – that is the way that they are made. Identical twins show closely similar levels of happiness.[14] The happiness of one twin is found to be a good predictor of the happiness of the other twin nine years later.

This can sound like bad news for those of us who are on the less ebullient side. There are at least two reasons why this is not as bad as it might appear. Firstly, the temperamental effect can have the advantage of providing a stabilising influence. One consequence is that negative events are less likely to derail our happiness.

One famous piece of evidence in this connection comes from an investigation entitled 'Lottery winners and accident victims: Is happiness relative?'[15] Briefly, it was found, as you would expect, that lottery winners enjoyed a surge in the happiness stakes, while accident victims experienced the reverse. However, over time, the surge and droop evened out, and the conclusion was that people generally reverted to their previous levels of happiness.

I think that this makes intuitive and experiential sense. Becoming chronically ill makes a dent in happiness, but then life goes on. There is other evidence though that with continuing health problems, reported happiness levels are, on average, just a fraction lower than for the general population.[16] Some reduction in taken for granted happiness would fit with my own experience.

But psychologists such as Nettle and Seligman also propose that there is considerable evidence that happiness can be 'worked at' and improved. This is the second reason why the temperamental constraint is not the final word. Happiness is about how we see ourselves and the world and, to some extent at least, we can learn to see these differently.

Happiness is a complex matter, but one fairly easily summarised piece of evidence is worth quoting. Fordyce, in 1987 developed a training program me to increase levels of happiness.[17] In comparison with a non-trained group, the programme succeeded in increasing reported levels of happiness. Moreover, this effect was maintained up to 28 months later. Interestingly, a more recent addition to the set-up has shown that adding in mindfulness training to the original programme, has produced a stronger 'happiness effect'.[18]

Overall then, I think that the messages in relation to managing depression and improving happiness are positive ones – it is possible. In this chapter I have given more space to the issue of managing depression. This is partly because for those of us who are chronically ill it may be the more urgent problem. It is also because the cognitive behavioural approach to coping with depression has been well established for quite a long time, and it is one that I have known about since before I got MS.

On the other hand, there has latterly been a spurt in psychological interest in happiness which has promoted renewed exploration on my part. One emerging consensus in these ideas is that happiness and depression are not simple opposites to each other. They seem to be independent, having different kinds of organisation and the involvement of separate causal factors. Therefore it is worth doing everything one can to avoid depression, but also, alongside that, there are advantages in trying, directly, to cultivate happiness.

Of course, Buddhists have been concerned with happiness for over 2,000 years and there is much to learn from the contributions they have made. The present Dalai Lama, in conjunction with a western psychiatrist has produced a book which specifically focuses on issues of happiness. This is *The Art of Happiness: A Handbook for Living* which is certainly worthy of consultation.[19]

Notes and References

1. Weihenmayer, E. (2001). *Touch the Top of the World.* London: Hodder and Stoughton. The quotation is from page 96.

2. Andrew, J. (2003). *Life and Limb.* London: Portrait.

3. One of these is Parkinson, B., Totterdell, P., Briner, R. B. & Reynolds, S. (1996). *Changing Mood: The psychology of mood and mood regulation.* Harlow: Addison Wesley Longman.

4. Parkinson et al. as above.

5. He has researched and published extensively. One of his books which is written for a more popular audience is Gilbert, P. (2000). *Overcoming Depression: A self-help guide using Cognitive Behavioural Techniques.* London: Robinson.

6. Sandovnick, A. D., Remick, R. A. & Allen, J. (1996). Depression and multiple sclerosis. *Neurology*, 46, 628-632.

7. Butler, G. & Hope, T. *Managing Your Mind.* Oxford: Oxford University Press.

8. The classic research in this area is by two psychologists called Duval and Wicklund. Duval, S. & Wicklund, R. A. A. (1972). *A Theory of Objective Self-Awareness.* New York: Academic Press.

9. I haven't come across any good accessible summary of Bandura's ideas. The original reference is Bandura, A. (1986). *Social Foundations of Thought and Action: A social cognitive theory.* Englewood Cliffs, New Jersey: Prentice Hall.

10. One of the many available introductions to Buddhist meditation and mindfulness is Weiss, A. (2004). *Beginning Mindfulness: Learning the way of awareness.* Novato CA: New world Library.

11. An accessible account of the development of this therapy approach is to be found in Segal, Z. V., Williams, J. M. G., & Teasdale, J. D. (2002). *Mindfulness Based Cognitive Therapy for Depression: A new approach to preventing relapse.* New York: Guilford Press. More information is available at the Centre for Mindfulness Research at the University of Wales, Bangor, www.bangor.ac.uk/mindfulness. Anyone interested in the developing interface between ideas about mindfulness and the practice of therapy would find it useful to investigate the work of Jon

Kabat-Zinn, on which Segal et al drew. His most recent book, Kabat-Zinn, J. (2005). *Coming to our Senses: Healing ourselves and the world through mindfulness.* New York: Hyperion, provides an account of his own development of Mindfulness Based Stress Reduction, and a useful overview of thinking about mindfulness in the Western context.

12. A more accessible account of mindfulness in relation to depression, directly addressed to anybody who is depressed is provided in Williams, M., Teasdale, J., Segal, Z., & Kabat-Zinn, J. (2007). *The Mindful Way through Depression.* New York: Guilford Press.

13. The details are Seligmann, M. E. P. (2003). *Authentic Happiness.* London: Nicholas Brealey Publishing, and Nettle, D. (2005). *Happiness: The science behind your smile.* Oxford: Oxford University Press.

14. Nettle, D. as above, p.92-93.

15. Brickman, P., Coates, D. & Janoff-Bulman, R. (1978). Lottery winners and accident victims: Is happiness relative? *Journal of Personality and Social Psychology,* 36, 917-27.

16. Nettle, D. as above, p.83.

17. Fordyce, M.W. (1977). Development of a programme to increase personal happiness. *Journal of Counselling Psychology,* 24, 511-21.

18. Smith, W. P., Compton, W. C., & West, W. B. (1995). Meditation as an ajunct to a happiness enhancement program. *Journal of Clinical Psychology,* 51, 269-273.

19. His Holiness the Dalai Lama and Cutler, H. C. (1998). *The Art of Happiness.* London: Hodder and Stoughton.

Chapter Eleven

High Days and Holidays

For many of us in the developed world in the twenty-first century holidays and outings provide enjoyable 'time out' from everyday lives. We spend time planning them in detail; we anticipate and look forward; we expect that the holiday itself will be interesting, exciting even, and, of course, enjoyable in complex kinds of ways. Afterwards we expect to take pleasure in recounting our experiences to friends and acquaintances.

The whole tourist industry, at home and world wide, is built around satisfying these needs. We are constantly reminded by advertisements, holiday brochures, Sunday newspaper supplements and travel books of all that is possible. We are told of all those places we must be sure to see before we die!

The advent of disability means that taking up these kinds of options becomes less easy. Of course, for everybody, there are constraints on taking advantage of desired travel possibilities. Having the necessary funds is the most obvious of these. If you are disabled a variety of extra challenges must be added in.

The Baby Bus...

It will have been evident that in my life before MS active outings and holidays were important, both to myself and to Pete. After MS the challenge has been to maintain that activity in some way. It will probably be clear that for us the solution has come to involve handcycles and tricycles.

But, these are bulky bits of equipment which are not easily transportable. For a while Pete managed the awkward task of getting the handcycle into the back of our rather tiny Renault Clio. For 'proper' cycling outings Pete manhandled my trike onto the roof of the Clio. His own bike was placed on a conventional rear bike carrier. The roof lift especially was rather demanding. Obviously we needed a more commodious form of transport, but it was not immediately apparent what would best suit our needs.

As we were beginning to contemplate better possibilities for transporting the handcycle we had a summer holiday on the Scottish west coast. This was a touring holiday for which we had hired a camper van. We took the handcycle and Pete's bike – we didn't at that stage have the trike. Although the camper van was obviously much larger than our Clio, there wasn't anywhere we could easily put the handcycle. It had to be somehow fitted into the bunk area above the cab.

The holiday was a very enjoyable one. It had been some years since we were last in Scotland. Tramping through the mountains is now impossible for us, but it still felt good to be among the hills and the west coast sea lochs again. The better views we had from the higher driving and passenger seats of the camper van were greatly apreciated, as was the luxury of having an 'on-board' loo. These days I can't easily manage the 'behind a bush' strategy, so finding an available loo out in lonely places can be a real problem and most unwelcome distraction from the real purpose of the outing.

Hence the advent of what we christened the 'day-van project'. Suitably adapted motor homes are a vehicle of choice for quite a number of disabled people, and after our holiday in Scotland we could see why.

Many camp sites now cater quite well for the needs of people with disabilities, and having 'mod-cons' to hand in the van certainly added to the convenience of vehicle based travel and exploration.

However, a live-in vehicle was not really what we wanted. Our aim was to have a suitable vehicle that would enable us to get to places where we could use our various bikes for more active exploration. Also, although my father in his eighties was still driving, we knew that there would be quite a few occasions when we would want to be out with my parents, and now also have the handcycle with us. This would not be possible in a camper van, in which passenger seating is usually limited.

The search was on for a suitable larger but flexible vehicle. After some thinking and some trials, we decided on a Volkswagen Caravelle. Flexibility derives from being able to remove the rear passenger seats when required, which enabled us to put both the tricycle and handcycle inside the van at the same time, very useful on those holidays where we've wanted to have both available. Pete's bike goes on a rack on the rear of the vehicle. For a while, after we had bought the tandem trike, we even managed to transport this inside the van, though eventually we decided that a trailer would be easier.

On first inspecting our new van, our American niece, Carys, announced with some amazement in her voice 'you have a bathroom in your car!' Actually it is just a Thetford chemical loo and a sink, but it solves the 'behind the bush' problem very nicely. The van is rather on the large side – hence its christening by some of our friends as the 'baby bus'. But it serves our current needs pretty well and it has taken us over 70,000 miles over the last six years.

Home Territory…

Using the tandem trike means that we are able to get out and cycle straight from our house. We are lucky to have quick access to reasonably quiet Cheshire lanes. On fine weekends we often take a short afternoon ride of around eight or nine miles, or else we go out over the lunch time period and stop for a pub lunch around mid-way. I thouroughly appreciate that we are able to do this. There is a feeling of freedom and exhilaration in being able to ride rather faster on the tandem trike than I can on my single trike. We are lucky to be able to get out so easily on to good cycling territory.

So, what do we class as 'home territory'? It goes a way beyond these outings from the house to include those places we can reach in an easy day trip. We continue to take advantage of our close proximity to the Peak District. The extended circular walks over the hills and through the dales, which we used to do, are no longer possible, but we have found various alternatives.

The Peak District would perhaps not initially appear to be the best place for easy cycling, but there are some accessible, and very beautiful cycling routes through the heart of the Peaks. These, as is so often the case, are the result of railway closures in the 1960s. The best of these are the 13 mile Tissington Trail and the 17 mile High Peak Trail which together provide around 30 miles of excellent cycling.

These trails are well surfaced and well maintained, and just as importantly they have no problematic barriers. There are gates but they open in both directions and, being on a strong spring, they are self closing and easily managed. They are exceptional in the sense that these rail lines were built at a high level and around the contours of the hills, rather than through the valleys. They provide wide and extensive views of the characteristic Peak District scenery – the patchwork of hillside fields, the dry stone boundary walls, and the trees on the skyline. There is also a colourful display of trail side wild flowers in the spring and summer months.

There are a number of other good old railway cycling trails within the boundaries of the national park, and a number of riverside paths which pass through the characteristic dales of the Peak District and provide good handcycling routes. On the northern outskirts of the park is what is one of the most spectacular handcycling routes anywhere. New Mills is a small Victorian mill town, but just behind the main road the buildings give way to what some regard as one of the most striking landscapes in urban Britain. The ground suddenly drops away into a deep gorge with the river Goyt at the bottom. This gorge was previously inaccessible, but now a new dramatic aerial walkway connects the existing pathways at either end. This Millennium Walkway is a graceful silvery steel structure resting on a series of columns standing on the edge of the bed of the river. Thus, the walkway is marvellously suspended part way up the side of the gorge. The more conventional riverside continuations at either end of the walkway make this a most enjoyable handcycling route.

Apart from enjoying the scenery and the activity, another pleasure gained from some of our Peak District outings is the ability to meet up with some old friends. Mary and Seamus live in Sheffield, so the Peak District provides a convenient and very pleasant context for a get together. Mary is an old school friend of mine from Aberystwyth, and we have all shared an enjoyment of walking and cycling over many years. Now, when we meet up, I handcycle and the others walk, though we have sometimes cycled together. Usually we meet for lunch, or afternoon tea and a good chat, when we can catch up on each other's lives. Then, before or after, we walk and continue to chat.

There is a partly urban connection in a different area which also allows easy day trips from home, but in the opposite direction from the Peak District. This is provided at Liverpool and the Mersey estuary, and the end of the Wirral peninsular. These are not where we would have gravitated in days gone by, but now we have found they provide us with good cycling routes for both handcycle and trike and they make a rather good contrast to the Peak District trails.

These paths are coastal or estuary ones and so naturally have the advantage for us that they are largely flat. The Liverpool route finishes up at the Albert Dock, having started off five miles up the Mersey estuary and being close to the water all the way. The views up and down the estuary and across to the Wirral are interesting and striking, even if not scenic in quite the conventional sense. One of the advantages of ending up at the Albert Dock is that there are places to eat for a half way rest, and various museums if one wants different kind of entertainment.

Enjoying the Flat Lands…

My reduced mobility has led us to explore parts of the country which we would have completely ignored in the past – the flat lands of East Anglia. Previously, I tended to dismiss this kind of area as being rather boring landscape-wise. But when we took our first holiday with my single trike, the flatter lands came to have a new attraction.

We rented a farm cottage in Norfolk just outside the small town (or maybe large village) of Reepham. It turned out to be a very attractive habitation with a large central square and an interesting church. It was conveniently placed for reaching most parts of Norfolk, being about 9 or 10 miles north of Norwich, about the same distance from the Broads, and a little further from the north Norfolk coast.

Much of our exploration was in the immediate area around and about Reepham, an excellent centre for cycling. My abiding memory of Norfolk is of quiet lanes, and views over ripe cornfields with masses of lovely red poppies along the field edges. So there were views – and often good ones. The hills were gentle – but sufficient to provide long and sweeping perspectives. It was the best place we could have found to try out my newly motorised trike. It was a huge pleasure to find that I was able to cycle again in what turned out to be interesting and attractive countryside.

We also investigated some of the towns and villages of the northern coast. The estuary and mud flats of Blakeney and Wells-Next-The-Sea provided a rather different kind of coastal landscape from that we are used to. When we visited Blakeney the tide was out so that we were able to find a path across the flats on which handcycling was possible. We returned along the muddy creek, with stranded small boats, which was the low tide estuary.

A holiday in the area also had the benefit of giving us another opportunity to visit our friends Marion and Panos. We make weekend visits to their Cambridge home on a reasonably regular basis. Marion is a fellow psychologist, whom I met when we were both doing post-graduate work at Lancaster University. Panos was there at the same time completing a master's degree in computing. Marion works as a clinical psychologist and has a particular focus on supporting children who are suffering from cystic fibrosis. We have a lot in common for all sorts of reasons, and their supportive friendship over the years, and especially since I got MS has been very important to me and us.

A later, different 'flat lands' holiday was our first visit abroad since the worsening of my MS. This was in the summer of 2001 when we decided that flat, cycle friendly Holland would make a good destination. Again, I don't think that this would have been on our holiday list in pre-MS days.

After some deliberation, we decided to head for the province of Zeeland, and in particular the peninsular of Walcheren. This is part of the 'dams and polders' landscape of south Holland, just north of the Belgian border, and within easy striking distance of Zeebrugge, to which we crossed on the overnight ferry from Hull.

It is effectively a delta area of islands and peninsulas divided by the estuaries of the river Scheldt. It was devastated by the North Sea storm surge floods of 1953, which also affected eastern England. Since then the huge Delta Project has completely altered the geography of the area. There are now thirteen dams constructed across the various estuaries, reducing the length of coastline open to the sea from 700 kilometres to just 25. Thus the landscape is very much man-made, but does have a dramatic quality of its own.

But what about the cycling? This turned out to be much more interesting and varied than we had expected. The dams provide quite impressive cycling routes. The Veerse Gat dam, for example, which adjoined Walcheren, has a broad road-width cycle 'path' along its top. From it there are extensive views down to the sand dunes and beaches of the North Sea on one side, and to the now freshwater Veerse lake on the other.

More traditional dikes circle around the Walcheren coast, and after the initial push up to the top, these also provide easy cycling with good sea views. The attractively wooded areas behind the coast offer a different kind of cycling experience. These paths are not tarmacked, but still of good cycling quality. They are somewhat akin to forestry routes in this country, although the woods are predominantly natural and deciduous.

As well as the countryside there were attractive old towns to visit in Zeeland. Some of the more noticeable features were steep roofed and many windowed town halls, and white painted balance beam bridges over the waterways. One of the towns to which we cycled, alongside the Veerse Meer was the 15th century Veere.

We made this ride on a Sunday and it was obviously a very popular route with the locals – positively teeming with cyclists. The town had purpose built bike parks, all with rows and rows of parked bikes. If this number of people had arrived by car, rather than cycle, the town would have been impossibly jammed up. As it was there was space to walk around in a leisurely way and enjoy the old buildings and a picnic on the lakeside.

An incident in the market square of another town reinforced the impression of how strongly cycling in Holland was integrated into everyday life and activities. A young woman crossed the market place in front of me – but somewhat perilously. She was pushing a bike with one hand, and a pushchair loaded with a small child and shopping with the other. She proceeded to lean the bike against a convenient wall, and then unload the shopping from the push chair onto carriers on the bike. She lifted the child onto the bike child seat. Next she folded the lightweight pushchair, and attached it to the side of the bike by means of an obviously purpose made fitting. She got on to the bike herself and pedalled away – shopping, with child, done, without any need for vehicular transport.

Coast and Waterside…

The approach to finding routes which are mostly easy in gradient terms adopted above was to look for countryside which is predominantly flat. Another tactic that has already emerged is to try to identify particular routes on which hills are not likely to be too long or demanding.

Our most successful ploy has been searching out coastal, lakeside or riverside routes. Of course such routes are not wholly flat, but they are often predominantly so, and they usually satisfy our other selection criterion of being scenicly appealing. We have explored some attractive parts of the British countryside which we might not otherwise have investigated, and re-examined other more familiar areas. The strategy has also been used in some exploration we have begun beyond the bounds of the British Isles.

On a summer holiday in North Devon we cycled most of the Tarka Trail. This is very much an estuary path along the Taw and Torridge rivers, but it is also a Sustrans ex-railway path, and so a nice well-surfaced trail. This is not altogether new territory for us. Pete was brought up in Croyde, about 12 miles north of Barnstaple. Croyde is now the rather noisy capital of the North Devon surfing scene, but in the fifties and sixties it was a quiet seaside holiday village.

We cycled north from Barnstaple to Braunton, along the river Taw. On another day we cycled south on the other side of the Taw, first to Fremington Quay, which had been an important station and port, and then on to Instow, across the river Torridge, from the old port and ship building town of Appledore. Riding along these trails gives a completely different, and much closer view of this estuary landscape than could ever be available from the road.

This is an excellent cycle path. It is a pity that almost impassable barriers on the northern Barnstaple to Braunton section diminished its appeal. The only way for us to manage them was for Pete to upend the tandem trike onto its two rear wheels, and then manoeuvre it around the barrier, not a very easy operation – the upended trike is quite unwieldy and difficult to manage. On a more recent visit to the area we have been very pleased to find that the barriers have been modified, and are now much more easily negotiable.

After the more serious advance of my MS and associated disability we did wonder whether we would still be able to make enjoyable visits to the Lake District, which had previously been a favourite weekend destination for us. I'm glad to say that, with a few adjustments, continued appreciation of this beautiful part of the country is possible. With a bit of effort we have been able to find quite a number of accessible routes – which are often alongside lakes or rivers.

Keswick has become one of our favourite destinations. It has an ideal position close to Derwentwater and with views of the hills and mountains all around. We have a favourite hotel, with views over the lake, to which we keep returning. The walk directly from the hotel, along the eastern shore of Derwentwater is a busy and popular one, but still one of which I never tire.

The views down the lake to the spiky Jaws of Borrowdale, across to the rounded switch back of Cat Bells, up above the path to the wooded cliffs of Walla Crag, and backwards to the looming bulk of Skidaw are hugely impressive, but change dramatically through different seasons, weather and light conditions. The path, thanks to the National Trust, is a good handcycling route with variable terrain – through woods, across streams, over grassy meadows. For the last part I abandon the handcycle to walk directly by the stony lake shore.

We have ridden all the way around the lake on the tandem trike – a distance of about 16 miles. For us this is a reasonably demanding ride with some moderate hills on the road along the western shore. But it is a beautiful ride along a fairly quiet road and now with impressive views over to the crags of the eastern side of the lake. The return road is busier, but usefully it is flatter, hugging the lakeside more closely.

There are also a couple of routes which can be handcycled, but which really give us a good feeling of being very much in among the mountains. From just near the village of Braithwaite, north of Derwentwater, there is a long valley following the Coledale beck. The track is reasonably wide and rises gently, leading to the old Force Crag mine. This is a quiet valley, away from the bustle around Keswick, and there are high hills and splendid views all around. Over the other top end of Derwentwater, from Threlkeld, it is possible to drive up to the Blencathra centre. Blencathra itself rises steeply up above, but onwards there is another valley side bridleway with an easy gradient. Again there are wonderful views and a splendid feeling of being right in the mountains.

A very different waterside visit was a city-based one. This was a long weekend visit, which we made in 2002, to the city of Stockholm. It was the first time we had taken a flight anywhere since the worsening of my MS, and so the first time we had taken the handcycle with us in this situation.

Stockholm is very much a watery place – it is built on fourteen islands at the junction of the Baltic Sea and lake Malaren. It is mostly pretty flat and access is good, so explorations by handcycle were no problem – we clocked up just about 25 miles in our three day weekend.

One of our most impressive visits was one made by most visitors to Stockholm. This was to the Vasa Museum, which has been constructed around the ship of that name, which briefly sailed across Stockholm harbour in 1628. The builders of the ship intended it to be the pride of the Swedish navy, but sadly a design fault meant that it was top-heavy and it sank on its maiden voyage. The Baltic sea has a low level of salinity and consequently the ship is well preserved. In 1961 it was successfully brought to the surface again. It is now circled by multiple walkways (also wheelchair accessible) so that one can view the ship from all sides and different heights, and inspect it now in all its glory.

In spite of the good access, we did find ourselves getting almost marooned as a consequence of having the handcycle. We made an afternoon visit to the extensive open-air Skansen Museum. This provides a hillside reconstruction of various clusters of old buildings from the Stockholm area – a whole ancient neighbourhood to explore. We spent a leisurely afternoon wandering around, stopping now and again to investigate the interiors of some of the buildings which were open for internal investigation.

According to a general guidebook we had purchased in the UK prior to our visit, the museum was open until 10 o'clock in the summer, so we thought we had plenty of time to wander around. But soon after five we began to see that the place was beginning to empty. We went back to the top of the hill with the expectation of riding the cog railway down to the bottom and the main entrance.

But the railway had stopped running so we had to make our own way to the entrance gate. Then we found that was closed too! There was a turnstile gate nearby which was obviously intended for late exiting – but how could we manage that with the handcycle? Fortunately a Swedish family in the same situation appeared. We were able to send them out with the front half of the handcycle, and Pete and I were just about able to get through with the wheelchair section – we were successfully out after a few uneasy moments

Pembrokeshire...

This Welsh county has been another important holiday destination for us – not just on one occasion but over quite a number of years, especially since I got MS. This is another coastal destination, indeed it is the only British national park which has been designated as such because of its exceptional coastal landscape. The special feature of the park is its long distance footpath that closely hugs the cliff tops. In days gone by we were able to take extended walks along these paths, but this is no longer possible. We have had to find other ways of enjoying the Pembrokeshire landscape.

Over the last ten years or so, towards the end of May we have taken a week's holiday in Pembrokeshire. In doing this we followed an established custom of my parents and one of my sisters. Pembrokeshire is especially attractive at this time of year, rather quieter than in the busy summer period, and when the beautiful wild flowers on the lane sides and cliff paths are at their best.

These holidays have given us a specially relaxed and enjoyable context in which to spend time with my parents. At the time that we first joined them on these holidays in 1998, my father was 83 and my mother was almost 84. Regardless of my physical abilities it was obviously not going to be a time for rushing around and taking strenuous walks.

Nevertheless, it was not a time for just sitting around either. My parents were fortunate, retaining both physical and mental capabilities well into their eighties. They continued to be able to take walks of a few miles or more, even if at a rather slower pace than in their younger years. I was glad that they could still get onto and enjoy the cliff walks in this way, but I cannot help feeling a serious degree of envy. They in their eighties could walk better than I could in my fifties! My challenge had to be to find ways in which I could still enjoy this landscape of cliffs and coves.

Part of the solution was to identify places where it is possible to get right onto, and even along the cliff tops with the handcycle. Over the years we have identified a surprising number of such places all along the path from Saundersfoot near the southern end to Newport bay in the north. Inevitably, some of these are of the less dramatic kinds. However, there are also places where it is possible to get access to the high cliffs which are at the heart of the Pembrokeshire experience.

Such access is available especially at the promontories of Lydstep Point and St. Govan's Head, but also at Stack Rocks. The topography of these areas is such that the land approaching the cliffs is unusually flat. Probably because of this all three areas are used by the military for training purposes. Walkers can only get there at specified times, but for me the little bit of required advance planning has the most rewarding pay-off.

On St. Govan's Head there is a surfaced track from the car park on to the broad, flat headland itself. This is a wide open area with a greatly spacious feel. The covering of short grass with very low stony outcrops allows easy and free handcycling. This is quite unlike the narrow, bounded and uneven paths of most of the coast path, but the views are the same. I can see dramatic and imposing cliffs stretching into the distance. I can also get quite close to the edges and look downwards at the rocks and changing sea below. These all provide a great sense of freedom and exhilaration. I feel that I am experiencing the essence of what the coast path is all about within this tiny part.

Another pleasure of these holidays has come from the various cottages in which we have stayed. Many of these have had positions very close to the coast and the path and have provided dramatic views along the coast or down to sandy bays. It is difficult to choose between places and cottages, but my overall favourite has been Glandwr cottage on the Parrog at Newport. Newport nestles beneath a Norman castle and the striking hill of Carn Ingli, a coastal outlier of the Preseli hills. The Parrog is the harbour area along the Nevern estuary at Newport.

Glandwr cottage is situated near the end of a single track lane which leads down to the estuary. Just a few yards down the lane outside the cottage, when the tide is out, there is access to the stony and rocky foreshore. Just a little further along you reach the road in front of the large houses, which once belonged to merchants and sea captains. The road then climbs very gently and becomes an accessible path, above low cliffs and a small sandy cove, still with the views across the estuary to the sand dunes on the other side.

Further along, the path becomes a cliff side route. To go further on I have to abandon the handcycle. There is a tricky (for me) but very short stretch of steep rocky path, worn smooth by the passage of many feet. There is a very big step and nothing to hold on to. In the narrow space it is impossible for anybody else to help. Keeping secure and keeping balance is difficult, I almost become a climber, and have to be really very careful about where I place my feet, but I do want to get further so take the risk.

Once this challenge is overcome, the cliff path becomes easier. Slowly, and with care, I can walk here. Our target is to achieve the grassy spot, where I can look straight down the steep cliff face to the kind of rocky cove which typifies the coastal path. In the Spring we expect to find patches of the lovely sky blue, star-like Squill flowers. These flowers are quite small, but a mass of them has a strong presence. There are also sea pinks and white sea campions and perhaps a stray bluebell here and there. This is a wonderful spot to sit and enjoy the views all around.

In May 2004 we had a marvellously restful holiday here, with blue skies and sunshine everyday. Pete and I would handcycle into

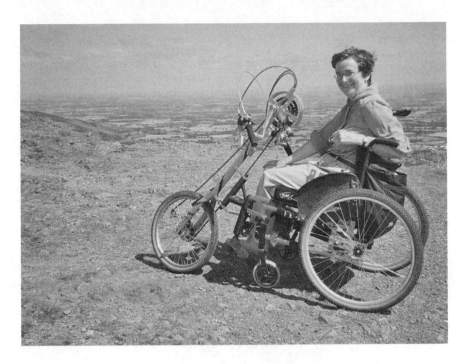

On the top – Worcestershire Beacon

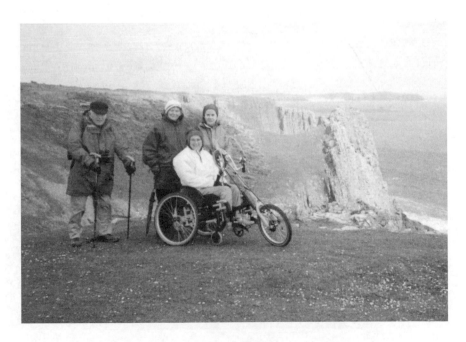

On the edge of the Pembrokeshire cliffs

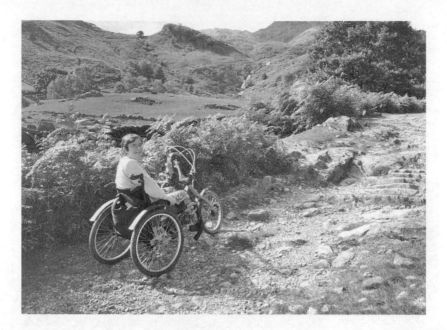

Above Grasmere

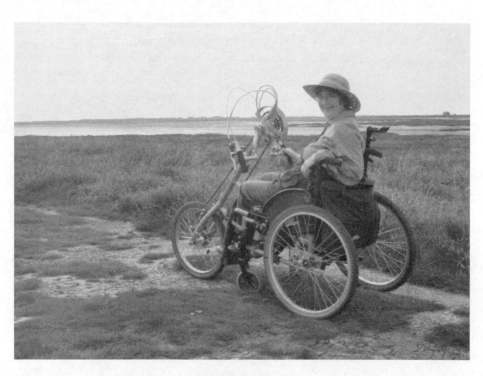

Norfolk flats

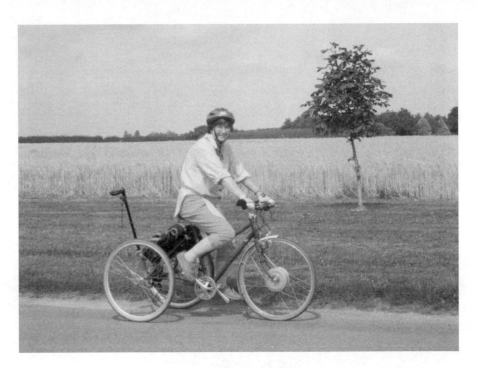

Triking in Norfolk

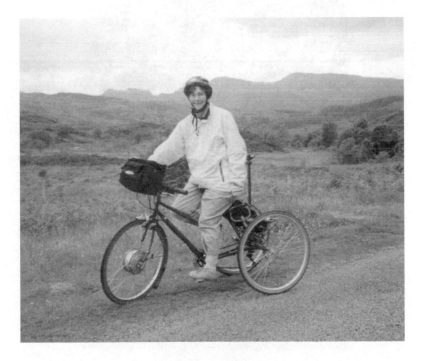

Towards the mountains

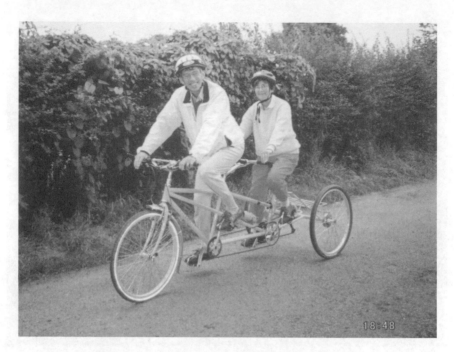

In the Cheshire lanes

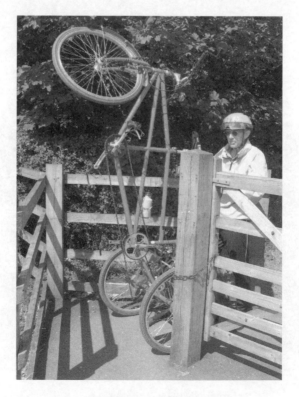

Trouble with barriers

Newport for some shopping, a browse around, and a cafe visit most mornings. In the afternoon we would all drive to somewhere near for a leisurely amble. During the week we had a quiet celebration of my mother's ninetieth birthday. Sadly this was to be our last holiday together. My father died the following February, a week short of *his* ninetieth birthday. We did, though, come back in 2005 with my mother and sister, and we were able to feel the sense of the presence of my father in the beautiful places that we had enjoyed together the previous year.

Visits to Aber…

My parents remained living in Aberystwyth through my father's retirement and for us it has been a good place to visit regularly through all the years of our marriage. We have been lucky that my parents lived in such a pleasant and attractive location.

The character of our visits necessarily changed somewhat with the advent and then worsening of my MS. There was a period when we had to drive the mile or so into town on a Saturday morning, something that we would never have done previously. The walk into Aberystwyth, then onto the promenade, with a leisurely wander around the town was a part of our weekend tradition. Having to use the car was not the same at all.

Having the handcycle has meant that we can, albeit in a slightly different way, reclaim the earlier tradition. Our usual circuit takes us along the Rheidol riverside cycle path and onwards to the harbour, though its days as a working port are long over. Nowadays, the more recently developed marina provides moorings for some opulent but also for some more restrained leisure sailing boats. The leftovers of a working fishing harbour are indicated by large piles of lobster pots often left on the harbour side wall. Beyond the harbour, and above the river Ystwyth lies one of the local hills – Pen Dinas – with ancient hill fort and monument to the battle of Waterloo on top.

From the south promenade, if conditions are right, we can see right down to the beginning of the Pembrokeshire coastline. The prom passes beneath the ruins of Aberystwyth castle. This is one of the castles built by Edward I to subjugate the Welsh. In its present condition it no longer rivals the coastal castles of North Wales, having come off badly in one of the civil war skirmishes. The prom turns a sharp corner and now, to the north, the outline humps and bumps of the higher parts of the Lleyn peninsular are often visible. Thus, on a good day, from this corner point, we can view the whole dramatic sweep of Cardigan Bay.

Around the corner comes our first view of Aberystwyth pier – somewhat battered, but still with a certain kind of attraction. On the right are the extensive neo-gothic buildings of the old college. Surprisingly they were built to be a hotel, rather than for educational purposes, at the cusp of Aber's popularity as a Victorian holiday resort. Beyond the pier the view extends along the main promenade. Now, multicoloured three to four storey traditional sea front hotels line the landward side, interspersed with more sober buildings (at least in outward presentation) which have been converted as student residences.

The northern end of the prom is marked by another hill – the English named Constitution Hill. A fellow South Walian once described Aberystwyth to my grandmother as that place with a coal tip at the end of the prom! This is really not justified, but one can see the basis for the intended insult. The underlying rock is shale, and on the seaward side collapsing shale, which might be seen as lacking attractiveness. But the hill taken in its entirety provides an imposing marker to the end of the prom and the town. It also provides, from the top, the beginning of an attractive cliff walk. I can no longer climb up there, but the Victorian funicular railway allows access to enjoy the excellent views up the coast.

Visits to Aber in the days before MS would have provided good walking opportunities, either immediately in the surroundings of the town, or a short car ride away. These days expeditions have to be shorter, but there are still quite a few available possibilities. Two favourites are seeing the feeding of the red kites, and the sand dunes at Ynyslas.

The red kite is a most attractive bird of prey, with an impressive wing span of around five and a half feet. In contrast to the broad wings of the buzzard, those of the kite are narrower. Its most characteristic feature is its fanned, forked tail. It has lovely markings in reddish brown and a mixture of paler colours, especially on the underside. It is a beautiful, almost elegant bird.

There was a time when it was very common in this country. It is very much a scavenger and it was often a resident of medieval towns, where there were good pickings, but by the middle of the last century its distribution had dwindled to very limited numbers in mid Wales. Over more recent years conservation and positive support have ensured that numbers have increased dramatically. Re-introductions at various centres mean that kites can now be seen across a number of areas throughout the British Isles.

One of the early support centres is at Nant yr Arian, a forestry area about 8 miles outside Aberystwyth. Food is put out for the birds regularly, every day of the year. Typically somewhere around thirty birds come and take advantage of this largesse. The birds wheel and soar around, sometimes diving down to get the best bits, on occasion with a degree of competition. With so many swooping around there are views of these beautiful birds from all directions, an impressive acrobatic display.

It is also at a very impressive location. The birds fly above a small, irregular pine fringed lake, approached down a short, steep hill to the lake and its stony edge. Sometimes we walk on to a second lake which gives more open, extensive views to the high hills of the Pumlumon range beyond. We return on the far side away from the lake. The path (still accessible) contours around, and up and down over a series of bumpy hillocks scattered with pine trees of varying sizes and with heather and whinberry bushes in the spaces. I have to work quite hard on the handcycle, but there will also be opportunities for me to swoop downhill. There are likely to be glimpses of one or two kites who have extracted themselves from the main throng over the lake.

A second favourite outing is to the estuary and sand-dunes at Ynyslas. The first approach into the sand-dunes is through soft sand which makes for rather difficult handcycling. A pusher here is essential! Fortunately, we soon reach a short board walk over the dunes which then becomes a hard shell based path – a reasonable handcycling surface.

Following on there is a flat area of dune slack, often with lying water. In the Spring, in both these areas there is a good display of flowers to be found in among the predominant marram grass. The lovely pink, creeping rest harrow contrasts with the bright yellow bird's foot trefoil. There is also yellow stonecrop, and the bright red of scarlet pimpernel if you look carefully.

Beyond the dune slack there are steps which climb up the higher dune ahead. This is where the handcycle is abandoned. Having avoided using my legs on the first part of the 'walk', I have enough energy to climb. Our target is a viewing platform at the highest point on the dunes, almost like reaching a hill top in that it provides the same kind of panorama of splendid views all around.

Northwards, across the estuary, are the water side buildings of the town of Aberdyfi. The substantial, pale painted houses show up strongly against the green of the hills above. Looking inland the view is towards the higher reaches of the Dyfi estuary – water or stretches of yellow sand, depending on the state of the tide. Beyond are the hills which overlook the estuary, often most striking when they look dark and brooding on an overcast day. Westwards to the sea, I can see the long stretch of beach, probably fairly empty even in the middle of summer. Here the water is likely to be rougher, with white breaking surf. Further down the coast is the linear beach side village of Borth, between the sea and the flat brown Cors Fochno behind. I am usually reluctant to leave these views and take the return path.

But what is there to do on a rainy day? Most likely we would visit the Aberystwyth Arts Centre, in the midst of the main university campus, on the third hill above the town. This provides grand and attractive spaces for different functions on three levels – cinema, theatre, great hall (for concerts and degree ceremonies), and various exhibition galleries.

On a wet Saturday afternoon we will almost certainly be able to find at least one exhibition that is of interest, browse in the book shop and look around the craft centre. At some point we will gravitate to the middle floor café, which has tables arranged along the wide and towering window spaces (up to the next floor). The seats provide extensive views over the town and sea below, and on one side to the first hills of the interior. It is a good place to relax and loiter, enjoy the views, and eavesdrop on the conversations around.

We are very lucky that visiting Aberystwyth still provides us with the opportunity to visit old friends. We often used to meet up with Mary and Seamus when our visits to see my parents coincided with Mary's visits to hers – and we would often attempt some co-ordination. Sadly, both of her parents have now died and so their visits to Aberystwyth are much rarer.

In the meantime some very old friends of ours, Dewi and Nerys, have conveniently moved to Aberystwyth. Dewi was one of Pete's first friends at Keele – forty years ago. And we've known Nerys for close to thirty years. Both of them are Welsh speaking and have spent all their working lives in Wales. Dewi was appointed deputy director of education in Ceredigion in 1995 and the family moved up from Carmarthen in 1996.

We had kept in close touch since Keele days, but it was a real bonus to have them living in Aberystwyth, and we make an effort to get together most times we are there – which is quite frequently. We meet for coffee at our favourite cafe in town, or for an evening meal, or we go over to their house just outside Aberystwyth. It is so good to be able to have that close and regular contact. They have been a real support to us, especially since the advent of MS.

More recently, some other friends have moved to the Aberystwyth area. These are Gaye and Colin. Gaye was a one time research fellow at Keele University and Colin lectured there in Education. Then Gaye got a post at Crewe+Alsager and joined the Independent Study team. She brought her specialist background and strong research experience in Health Studies. In 1992 she became head of the department in which Independent Studies was placed. Later still, in 1995, she became my PhD supervisor. Having a friend as one's supervisor could have been a risky situation, but Gaye was a good supervisor and we are still friends.

Gaye has had a long time connection with the village of Borth, having had a holiday cottage there for many years. On retirement she and Colin have bought a house which is spectacularly positioned at the top end of Borth, high up and with marvellous views down over the village and Cors Fochno, across the sea to the Lleyn peninsular, and inland up the Dyfi estuary. So now we can visit and enjoy these, talk over old times at Crewe+Alsager, and catch up with news of ex-colleagues.

A Degree of Restriction?

Walking in the countryside is a hugely popular recreational activity. For many it provides an important antidote to the pressures of everyday life. We can get away from things into the open air and in beautiful surroundings. Being able to stride along gives a sense of physical freedom. We know that the exercise is good for us. We may well become tired, but with this tiredness there will also be feelings of accomplishment and of psychological well-being. Becoming disabled means that the ease and taken for granted quality of this activity is lost. Even if we can walk a little, the easy rhythm and flow is no longer available to us. It is all a great deal more laboured.

The attractions of being out in the countryside remain, but support for access is required. I am most fortunate that my handcycle allows me to get actively out and into the countryside. I know very well that handcycles are expensive and so not readily affordable by everyone. Usefully, handcycles are available for hire at a few country parks and such places in some parts of the country. It would be of great benefit if a good choice of high quality mobility equipment was more widely available and publicised.

Another way to help people with disabilities enjoy the countryside is the provision of good routes without barriers. Things are improving partly as a consequence of the Disability Discrimination Act, but also resulting from pressure from those directly involved. Most National Parks now provide at least some access information and many are making an effort to reduce barriers. Pembrokeshire National Park, for example, has organised the removal of 300 stiles over the last ten years. The North Yorkshire Moors National Park is removing difficult gates and stiles and is aiming to open 25% of its bridle ways and 8% of its paths for easy access.

However, compared with able-bodied walkers, there is a shortage of information. The ordinary walker can select from a whole host of books and magazines which will give guidance on paths and suggested routes in all parts of the country. Apart from the various National Park booklets I only know of one published book which describes routes for people with disabilities. This is *Walking on Wheels* by Eva McCraken, which describes 50 wheel-friendly trails in Scotland.[1]

Another set of books which are 'wheel friendly' in a different kind of way, are those containing All Terrain Pushchair Walks, published by Sigma Leisure and which cover most of the National Parks.[2] Pushchairs are lighter and more easily lifted around obstacles in comparison with wheelchairs and handcycles, and certainly scooters, but there is still some common ground in relation to route requirements. Pete and I have certainly found some useful route ideas from these books.

Co-ordination is potentially of great importance. A body that has already provided some oversight in this area, and potentially could provide more, is the Fieldfare Trust.[3] The Fieldfare Trust is a charity which has the aim of improving access to the countryside for people with disabilities.

An important achievement has been the provision of access criteria for different countryside conditions. Through the Millennium Miles Project they have identified paths through the country which have a very high degree of accessibility. But because of their high quality in terms of accessibility the number of miles which reach this standard is quite small. We need information about paths which are reasonably accessible, but are more challenging. The Fieldfare Trust is hoping to work towards the internet recording of routes of this kind. Such an achievement would be ambitious but should be feasible using modern technology. Finding good accessible paths is difficult. For Pete and I finding a new path that is accessible and takes us to and through beautiful places is a cause for celebration: there is a sense of accomplishment – even triumph.

There is another, very different kind of restriction, that now characterises our holiday experience. We haven't taken much advantage of those cheap flights, or the more extensive long haul possibilities which are now available. We've hardly flown anywhere very much over recent years. Unlike the walking restrictions, these flying limitations have been more voluntary, more chosen.

We could, indeed, have flown to some far flung destinations. However, there is still the issue of what to do when we get there. We cannot readily take the trike, and especially the tandem trike, by air. We have taken the handcycle, and I expect that we will do so again. I'm sure that there are other cities besides Stockholm that we could explore in this way. I would also like to try taking the handcycle to a Greek island, or to the Portuguese Atlantic coast to see how we would get on. However, even with the internet, it is still difficult to get information about accessible possibilities in foreign parts.

There are other perspectives on this flying business. I certainly do not miss the tensions and potential delays of the airport experience. Increasingly, being 'dropped into' a new country does not feel like a good way to travel. Also, worries about the environmental effects of air travel have magnified enormously. For us this is something which we will continue to take into account when deciding about travel arrangements. Ferries, and perhaps trains, now have greater positive attraction for getting to foreign parts. There are plenty of European destinations left to explore in this way.

But restrictions can also provide benefits. One of the positive consequences of my having MS has been that we have spent more of our holiday time exploring various parts of the UK. As I've said we've visited and enjoyed some areas that we might have otherwise ignored. Overall, we feel that we've gained a better appreciation of the great variety of marvellous British landscapes. And there is still a great deal to explore. We want to spend more time in the Scottish Highlands and islands, and somehow, so far, we've managed to ignore Ireland altogether. There is plenty left to enjoy without leaving these shores. Some restriction, yes, but there are also lots of opportunities.

Notes and References

1. McCracken, E. (2006). *Walking on Wheels: 50 wheel friendly trails in Scotland*. Dumfermline: Cualann Press.
2. For example, Irons, R.&R. (2003). *All Terrain Pushchair Walks: North Lakeland*. Wilmslow: Sigma Press.
3. www.fieldfare.org.uk

Chapter Twelve

Disabled Body but Positive Self?

Bodily Ills and Mysteries...

The story I have been telling has focused very much on my psychological experience and coping in relation to my MS. Apart from mobility issues, physical aspects have been less centre stage. Now that I have had MS for quite a long time it seems worth looking backwards to comment on how things have changed in bodily terms over that time. In some ways they haven't recently been changing too much. One of my common answers to the perennial 'How are you?' question is the somewhat boring 'Pretty much the same'. Boring maybe, but I know that I am very lucky that I can answer in that way.

To what extent has my own disease progression coincided with, or differed from, expectations? Previously, I described how MS falls into two main forms. One involves the experience of successive periods of relapse and remission; the other is primarily progressive in character with things gradually getting worse.

So, how has it been for me? Early on, as described, I had quite a good period of remission after the initial relapse. But, then, after the next slow relapse, I eventually had to accept that there wasn't going to be any real remission experience. However, I haven't experienced, so far anyway, that expected continuing decline which should be part of progressive MS.

In fact, there has been some, if very small, improvement during the few years onwards from around 1998. It means that I don't fall down any more and my balance has improved to a degree. I can walk a little further than I could when things were at their worst. Most importantly, as I've reported, I can ride my tricycle again. These improvements have, so far, been maintained. They are certainly not dramatic, and I suspect that if I hadn't been monitoring my physical capabilities quite carefully, I might have missed them. So it can be beneficial to not always believe the rules for your disease, keep active, and keep an eye out for improvement.

My other departure from the 'rules' came before I even knew that I had MS. There was a period of around two to three years in the mid 1980s when I had a rather painful time with trigeminal neuralgia. The right side of my face was acutely sensitive to any kind of touch – washing and teeth cleaning were really difficult. When I walked, and as I put a foot to the ground, pain would jar upwards, especially into my head. I had frequent stabbing pains near the corner of my eye.

I went back and forth to the doctors but they couldn't make any suggestions as to where the problem had come from – just that it was one of those medical problem areas that was poorly understood. Although not that long ago, this was still before it was easy to check up one's symptoms on the internet. I took tegretol pills, which is the usual treatment. They didn't make the pain go away, but they did 'damp it down' and make it more bearable. Eventually it gradually faded away, and hasn't returned, although just occasionally I get a slight twinge or two.

When I got the MS diagnosis, someone lent me the appropriate major medical textbook. I read a bit of it and found that trigeminal neuralgia was sometimes a symptom of MS. However, the expectation was that this would occur after considerable progression of the disease and after a serious degree of de-myelination had taken place. When I told my consultant about my experience of having trigeminal neuralgia, his immediate response was a rather accusatory, 'Who told you that?' – as though I had invented the diagnosis for myself. To be fair, it doesn't quite fit with the supposed 'rulebook'.

There was a time when there was an unwillingness to accept that pain was a part of the MS experience. Now it is acknowledged that nerve pain does occur for many people as part of their MS. Pain is also a significant part of many other chronic illnesses. Rheumatoid arthritis comes to my mind as one such disease where pain is an unrelenting and regular part of experience.

Such pain is difficult to treat with conventional pain killers. Increasingly, psychological approaches to pain management are being seen as important, and have been pioneered, as part of a multidisciplinary approach, in various pain management clinics. I have been lucky that my own nerve related pain has not returned in any serious way. I get the occasional twinge in the right side of my face. I get more frequent pains down my left side, but these don't last long. Compared with many, I have nothing much to grumble about in this respect. For me, though, there is another kind of bothersome pain which is a less direct product of my MS.

There are other bodily functions which people normally take pretty much for granted but which can often become problematic in the context of disability and chronic illness. There is also the problem that they can be difficult to talk about easily and openly. In the past I mostly assumed that my bowels would work without my having to think about it too much. I could get constipated on holiday sometimes which was annoying, but it would usually right itself without too much trouble. But no longer. Now getting constipated is a perennial risk which I have to take considerable care to avoid.

The problem is that the desired end of easy and regular bowel activity seems difficult to achieve. This is frustrating because I really do all the recommended things. I am quite a fruit and veg junky. I consume extra fibre in addition. I snack on prunes and figs. I suspect that my daily exercise achievements are a great deal better than many able bodied people. But I still have a problem!

I need to resort to laxatives. I have tried out most of these. The problem is that the stronger ones give me 'gut ache' while the others are often ineffective. In any case, one worries about resorting to these since the packet always has the dire warning that their regular use is not desirable since it might ultimately make the whole problem worse.

The pain can be quite bad. It has the habit of appearing around 4 o'clock in the morning! Once the pain has started up it usually lasts, in an on–off fashion for several weeks. I usually get a couple of bouts, each lasting two or three hours, per day. A further frustration is that the medics do not seem to have any easy solutions either. If there was an offer of a magic wand to remove just one of my MS problems, I think that I might well choose to have no more problems with the functioning of my bowels ever again.

The other b. problem is with bladder function, though this has proved generally easier to manage. Mind you, in common with many people who have MS, I feel somewhat resentful to have two, seemingly opposite problems here. On the one side is the over-active bladder that can lead to a little bit of leakage at inappropriate times. On the other, there are those occasions, especially if I am under a bit of stress, when it is difficult to get the process to start.

Here, fortunately, there is a neat and easy medical solution which it took me a little time to pick up the courage to try, but which I would now recommend to anyone who finds themselves with this difficulty. This is self-catheterisation, which is much less fearsome than it sounds. Single use sterile, lubricated catheters are available in a foil pack. Basically, they comprise a plastic tube open at both ends. One end is inserted into the appropriate orifice which really does get quite easy after a little practice, and, behold, the yellow liquid runs out of the other end – quite a neat operation once one gets used to it.

The risk of leakage problem is taken care of with modern, highly absorbent pads which are readily available these days in most supermarkets. I know that many people feel there is considerable stigma associated with any kind of incontinence problem. I cannot see that there is any reason to be ashamed. A degree of embarrassment maybe, and it can be a nuisance and inconvenient. In actuality, though, it is a common problem, especially for women, and not just for the elderly.

Another common problem in MS and some other chronic illnesses, most especially ME, is that of fatigue. This is fatigue like you have never known it before. It is not like ordinary tiredness. I can sometimes feel after having walked half a mile as though I have walked twenty. It really can seem pretty impossible to put one foot properly, and in control, in front of the other. What is more annoying and frustrating for me is that I can sometimes get this feeling of exhaustion when I really don't think I have done anything. When I stop and think about it I realise I have been standing up for longer than I have realised. For me weight bearing of any kind seems to be crucial, because cycling has a more delayed effect. Getting tired is pretty frustrating, but I know that overall in this fatigue business I have got off pretty lightly.

A threat that I have been loath to think about, or accept that it could effect me, is one that is physical but also psychological. This is what is generally referred to as cognitive loss. MS leads to a reduction in the speed and ease with which messages are passed along neurones. This obviously effects physical responses and bodily processes, but it has become clear that it can also effect cognitive processes.

Most authorities now accept that MS influences cognition. It has the potential to lead to cognitive deficits such as short term memory problems, memory retrieval difficulties, problems in following a complicated storyline or in planning for the future. I find it difficult to contemplate that this could be happening to me. My cognitive, intellectual capability is an important part of who I am.

Fortunately, as with most MS symptoms, the incidence of such deficits is quite variable so I can continue to hope I might largely escape. At the same time the now unavoidable awareness of the prevalence of Alzheimer's disease means that I am certainly not alone in worrying about vulnerability to such effects.

I am aware that my memory is not as good as it was. On the other hand, I know this is also true of many of my age mates. We have reached that time in our lives when normal ageing begins to have some impact on memory in particular. The 'it's on the tip of my tongue' feeling becomes more prevalent for all of us. Consequently, I feel less singled out by any difficulties of this kind that might result from having MS, and have become more acceptant of this particular MS risk.

Being chronically ill leads to greater interaction with the medical profession than might have occured otherwise. I have had my share of consultations over the years that I have had MS. It is my GP who has been my most important source of ongoing advice and support. I have been fortunate that my doctor has combined both old fashioned and modern GP virtues, being a good listener with the best non-verbal communication skills. The consultation really is a consultation in that he discusses rather than imposes treatment possibilities. In the chronic illness situation that is most important.

Threatened Identity or a Quality Life?

My body and my relationship with my body have clearly changed. But I am more than my body. To what extent have *I* changed? Am I the same person I used to be? Change is clearly part of life – we all change. Does becoming ill and disabled lead to greater change than that which is part of life's ordinary progression? This issue is clearly of interest to those of us who have become disabled.

It is also an issue that has been of considerable interest to social scientists. Some kind of direct or implied reference to 'threatened identities' has been common. This is demonstrated in the titles of academic articles: 'Chronic illness as biographical disruption' and 'The genesis of chronic illness: narrative reconstruction'.[1] Most explicit and most extreme has been an article by Kathy Charmaz entitled, 'Loss of self: a fundamental form of suffering in the chronically ill'. She comments further that,

> ...*chronically ill persons frequently experience a crumbling away of their former self images...Affected individuals commonly not only lose self esteem, but even self identity...the person can no longer claim identities based on prior external activities. They are gone.*[2]

The issue of threats to identity is an important one, but this particular article made me quite angry and I have a number of objections to it. Firstly, for an academic article, the language is rather loose and woolly, and terms are not well defined. As I tried to explain early in this book, the concepts of self and identity are complex and multifaceted. Charmez does not do a great deal to explain her use of the concepts. Can identities be lost and completely 'gone'?[3]

There are plenty of examples where disabled or chronically ill people have worked to counter the threats and disruptions they face. Christopher Reeve was disabled to an extreme degree, but clearly it still gave him pleasure to reflect back over his previous acting career, and he made the huge effort to get back into the acting arena through becoming involved in directing a film.[4] Well, of course, Christopher Reeve was a fairly exceptional individual, and also with exceptional resources and contacts. A more ordinary example is the climber Jamie Andrew who went climbing again despite his loss of hands and feet.

A second important concern is the way in which Charmaz's research was carried out and the kind of conclusions drawn. The research drew on in-depth interviews with 57 respondents having chronic illnesses and disabilities. These respondents constituted an opportunity sample, that is they were people she could conveniently get access to. Thus, she could not be sure that her sample was representative and typical of the larger group from which it was drawn, and was made up of individuals who were quite severely ill and disabled.

Even so, she makes no attempt at all to qualify her conclusions. She refers in her title to a 'fundamental form of suffering' The implication appears to be, and nothing is said to contradict this, that such suffering is an inescapable part of being chronically ill. I do not think that such a conclusion is in any way justified on the basis of the limited evidence provided.

The identity focus is an important one in our attempts to understand change and development in chronic illness and disability. A slightly shifted approach recently used by social scientists, but which has now been fully adopted in everyday discourse, relates to quality of life. A good quality of life involves a subjective experience of well-being and general life satisfaction. To what extent can this be maintained when one becomes ill and disabled?

I'd like to describe another piece of research which is important because it provides a major contrast to that reviewed above. As with Charmaz's research, the title almost says it all. This second investigation is entitled 'The disability paradox: high quality of life against all the odds.' [5]

This research was also largely qualitative in character, but does provide some percentage indicators of main responses. Greater care has also been taken over the selection of respondents. Just over one hundred and fifty individuals from the Chicago metropolitan area were interviewed and this represented a 92.8% response rate of those contacted, which is exceptionally high. 93% reported that their disability had a moderate or serious effect on their lives and they are described by the researchers as having limited incomes and benefits, as having serious limitations in the activities of daily living, and being relatively socially isolated.

Quality of life is itself a complex concept and has been assessed in a number of ways, most usually self report questionnaires. These often include a health related component which might well be biasing in this context. In this research participants were asked to respond to an open question – 'In general how would you describe the quality of your life?' This could obviously draw on health aspects but did not draw attention to this aspect of life.

So, how do these respondents, who have serious and persistent health and disability problems, respond to this question? The disability paradox, as the researchers see it, is that very many report that they experience a good or excellent quality of life. The actual proportion affirming this was 54.3%. It is not possible to include many respondents' comments on their experience here, but a couple can provide an indicator: "Other people can't understand why I am so happy. They don't have the same appreciation of life. They would have to understand the satisfaction of using all my resources to conquer each day of challenges," and, "I don't like the way my disease is going but I can't complain. I have good days and bad days but all in all I have a good life."

One of the important points made in this research is that, although external observers might well think that people with disabilities and chronic health problems have a poor quality of life, many of those in this situation are able to focus on those aspects of their lives which are positive. There is a difference, perhaps a contrast, between the internal and external perspective. It seems to me that Charmaz, despite her qualitative approach, has found it difficult to fully appreciate this disabled perspective. She certainly seems to sometimes interpret a respondent's comments in a negative way when a different positive interpretation appears to be just as possible.

The third investigation considers both quality of life and identity issues. Again the title is instructive and worth quoting. It is, 'Sticking jewels in your life: exploring women's strategies for negotiating an acceptable quality of life with multiple sclerosis.'[6] This is another qualitative study which involves in depth interviews of 27 women volunteers who had had MS for mostly quite substantial periods of time (average 14 years). The overall aim of the research was to try to understand the strategies and tactics used to try to live an acceptable life when one has MS.

In this case the researchers might be criticised for taking a stance which involves looking for the positive, but the researchers show that they were well aware of the negative constraints of the disease. For many of the women interviewed, mobility problems and fatigue in particular had interfered with previous interests and activities, and all but one had retired from full-time work.

In the accounts of their experiences, the metaphors of 'battling', 'fighting' and 'struggling' are important ones for these women. The interweaving of both positive and negative experiences is an essential part of their adaptation to chronic illness. One respondent pictured her life as, 'A tapestry with some dark and dirty threads and some sparky ones'. Coping with MS can never be a static achievement. Such continuing adaptation requires considerable effort and resourcefulness.

Some of this effort is directed towards the maintenance of personal goals and a continuing sense of self and identity. Many women report that they are able to adapt and use previous job skills in their current more constrained, lives. Some have taken the opportunity to revive old interests – even if in an adapted kind of way. Thus a degree of continuity supports a sense of ongoing identity. For some, there may even be the possibility of greater freedom. One respondent described her pre-MS job as being pretty much seven days a week with time for nothing else, but that, 'MS has enabled me to open up my life in so many different directions'.

One of the other themes in the womens' comments is that of valuing and promoting positive moments rather than taking them for granted.

The researchers report that the conscious savouring of positive experiences contributed to a positive quality of life. Respondents comment on trying to squeeze in as many pleasurable activities as possible when times are good. Positive memories and the hope that such experiences will be repeated can help to maintain morale in more difficult periods.

This study is not an evaluation of how well people cope with chronic illness. It is a descriptive but rich account of determined efforts to make the most of difficult life-circumstances. It is an account with which I can easily identify, and one that is inspiring. Although the investigation is specifically about coping with MS, many of the coping responses would probably also be relevant to other chronic illnesses.

Narrative Coping...

Disability and chronic illness undoubtedly pose a threat to one's view of oneself and one's sense of identity. But the study briefly outlined above reinforces my own experience that such a threat is frequently resisted. Charmaz's conclusion that there is 'loss of self' is an oversimplification of the dynamic process of continuing struggle and adaptation.

There are good psychological reasons why we are likely to continue this struggle. Some of the pertinent ideas were discussed earlier in this book – in the second chapter. One such idea is that of self actualisation which was put forward by Carl Rogers. His position was that all of us, even in difficult times and circumstances, are motivated to move forward in our lives, and make the most of ourselves and our skills and abilities.

For me one of the most important contributors, whose theory supports our tendency to try to maintain a continuing sense of identity, is Seymour Epstein.[7] His approach, described earlier, can, as he puts it, be represented as a theory of a theory. He proposes that each person's self is seen as the personal theory which the person has about themselves and their place in the world. All of us need such theories in order to make sense of our personal experience and place in the world. Without such a theory our lives would be chaotic and confused. Thus, Epstein argues that we have a strong motive to maintain our implicit self-theories. In other words, there is a psychological impetus for us to retain our theory of who we are and our sense of identity.

But there is a problem. If such personal theories are to work effectively they cannot be static and unchanging. Our lives and experiences change. If our theories of ourselves are to stay effective they must change also and stay in tune with reality.

Ideally, these changes and adjustments are gradual – bit by bit. Part of Epstein's theory explains how such gradual change can best take place. Those of us who become ill and disabled have the problem that the changes that we face in our lives may well be quite considerable and quite sudden. Understandably, this can provoke quite a serious crisis of confidence and identity for some of us. But it is just as likely that many of us will struggle to retain, at least to some degree, our sense of self and identity.

Another aspect of the earlier discussion of self in chapter two is relevant here. The dominant view which psychologists now have of the nature of self is that it is complex and multifaceted. We manage our lives through a whole set of self-schemas which relate to the various self-relevant qualities and experiences. We have multiple identifies which relate to different experiences and contexts. There is a sense in which this multiplicity makes us more resilient. We can change some aspects of our views of ourselves without the whole system collapsing.

A different way of thinking about these processes of self-change is in terms of personal narrative.[8] As we tell our ongoing stories about ourselves, we are, by the nature of things, incorporating into them our changing experiences and changing lives. Telling the stories provides one way of accommodating ourselves to those changes. I do not wish to imply that making these changes and adjustments is easy and straightforward for those of us who face illness and disability within our lives. What I do want to suggest is that many of us will work at making the changes to our lives and ourselves – rather than just giving up.

The Self-Management Challenge...

Maintaining an ongoing sense of self and identity is important. But in addition we need to manage day to day psychological life: emotions and moods, worries and uncertainties, goals and rewards and so on. The idea of self-management is crucial within the world of work. In order to be successful one needs to have good skills in this area.

Effective self-management is also of value within the personal and psychological context. Ultimately this is what many self-help books are about. One book I have already mentioned, and which examines the psychology of self-management for the ordinary reader from a psychological base is *Managing Your Mind* by Gillian Butler and Tony Hope.

Previously, that is before the onset of my MS, I took my own psychological self-management pretty much for granted. Of course, there were less good days, various dissatisfactions and disappointments, and sometimes the experience of lowered mood. But on the whole I would have counted myself as pretty happy, and remarkably fortunate in my personal life, with a positive sense of day to day control.

Getting MS has undoubtedly made life more difficult. There are these unpleasant bodily symptoms which keep making their presence felt. My ability to get out and about in the way that I would wish is restricted. And, of course it just never goes away. So now more effort is required to maintain positive mood, to set realistic goals and to feel comfortable in this different life.

In a sense this book has been an exploration of managing my mind in these new circumstances, that is as a person with a disabling chronic illness, written from a psychologist's viewpoint. Has being a psychologist made any difference to my own coping? There is a sense in which the answer is in the negative. The kind of sense meant is that quite clearly you do not have to be a psychologist in order to cope well with the challenge of being chronically ill and disabled. As I've briefly demonstrated in passing, there are many non-psychologists who cope magnificently with greater, more severe disabilities than I have encountered.

On the other hand, I consider there are ways in which being a psychologist has eased my coping path. My psychological knowledge has provided me with a framework of understanding. This understanding has helped me to cope with difficulties, and to identify positive management strategies. My awareness of relevant books and articles has also enabled me to re-read useful contributions. I have also known how and where to seek out new and recently published articles.

There are many ways in which becoming ill and disabled means a loss of control. There are physical symptoms about which I cannot do a great deal. The progression of MS, and other chronic illnesses cannot be readily controlled – that is why they are chronic. But feelings of being in control of at least some aspects of our lives make an important contribution to psychological well being. Feeling that I am taking some psychological control over my life has been very important. The things that I do in this respect matter, and have consequences. Although they cannot have any effect on making the disease go away, they can help me to feel that there are ways in which I am in charge of my life.

Also, such feelings of taking psychological control in difficult and challenging circumstances, provide a sense of positive achievement. I'm doing well and being successful despite the problems that I face.

In a sense, I am making the kind of interpretations which turn an adverse situation to my advantage. This is a useful way of bolstering self-worth. It is a psychological tactic of considerable benefit.

I would be pleased if this book could aid readers in considering the value of self management processes. For those with a chronic illness there is an important source of help. The Department of Health now supports the Expert Patient Programme based on locally available Chronic Disease Self-Management Courses. These last for six sessions and are run as small structured learning groups of around a dozen or so people. The trained leaders will themselves have had experience of chronic illness. Courses should now be available in most localities. In many ways the programme fits with the spirit of this book.

Being Positive about Positive Psychology...

In its modern form psychology is still a relatively young discipline. But as I've tried to indicate, psychology has changed in the years since the beginning of my own involvement with the subject, and it continues to do so at quite a rapid rate.

One recent development which has attracted my attention and interest is the emergence and increasing influence of positive psychology. The emergence was marked by a special edition of the *American Psychologist* (a primary journal of the American Psychological Association) published appropriately in the millennium year of 2000.[9] This special edition focused wholly on positive psychology. In 2002 the large *Handbook of Positive Psychology* (over 800 pages and 50 contributors) was published.[10] This handbook demonstrated the substantial progress made in this developing area. A number of similarly large volumes, together with many journal articles have been published since. Fortunately, for the general reader, there is also a smaller, more accessible volume – the suitably named *Positive Psychology in a Nutshell.*[11]

So what is positive psychology? In the areas of psychology concerned with individual personal functioning and personal adjustment, there has been a tendency to focus on malfunctioning, what is going wrong, on a disease model – rather than on positive adjustment. The positive psychology approach argues that a shift of perspective is required. We need to give more attention to positive well being and successful functioning, even under difficult circumstances. Significant words from the titles of contributions to the Handbook give an indication of some of the topics that are of interest: hope, compassion, gratitude, humour, authenticity, happiness, love, altruism.

In the past, such topics would not have been considered amenable to empirical investigation. They would therefore have been seen as outside the accepted remit of academic psychology. Of course, as is usual in discipline change, the emergence of positive psychology is not something that happened completely out of the blue, around the year 2000. There have been earlier pioneering efforts – most notably in the work of Carl Rogers and the humanistic psychology movement during the nineteen sixties. These ideas were important, but, as indicated previously, they did not attain central acceptance and influence within the discipline. But in the late eighties and nineties there was a gradual accumulation of contributions which are now recognised as building the foundation of positive psychology.

What has positive psychology got to do with coping with disability and chronic illness? Does it have any relevance? For me it definitely does. I get information, understanding and inspiration from some of the research and theorising which has already taken place – and hope for more in the future. Some of the ideas which have already informed this account have been derived from positive psychology sources.

Positive psychology uses the resources of the discipline to investigate the nature of successful functioning. In the particular context of chronic illness and disability, the first thing to appreciate is that, although this state inevitably presents us with difficult challenges, many people do cope well, and manage their lives effectively. The task of positive psychology is then to obtain a better understanding of how this is achieved.

Timothy Elliot, with various colleagues, has researched into adjustment after spinal cord injury. In the *Handbook of Positive Psychology* he presents an overview of his and other people's work. His article is titled 'Positive growth following acquired physical disability', and it is one which is both interesting and inspirational.

Elliot makes the case that positive functioning and adjustment are certainly possible after disability has entered people's lives. But, more than that, he suggests that individuals can progress beyond their previous levels of functioning and adjustment. Disability can serve as a stimulus which leads us to see ourselves and the world differently. Elliot writes that

> ...*persons who have developed greater acceptance of disability will demonstrate a sense of meaning in their circumstances, value their selfhood, and maintain positive beliefs about themselves...individuals who incur a physical disability may do more than "survive" their condition; their resilience and clarity of purpose may result in a greater resolve for pursuing personal goals and an attainment of spiritual awareness and psychological adjustment that surpasses their previous level of adaptation.*[12]

Investigating the conditions that are conducive to the development of such positive adjustment then becomes an important research aim.

On the Other Side...

But how can we carry out such demanding research? Much earlier in this book I made some comment on the methods of research used within psychology and the social sciences. As I said, there is some disagreement about the most appropriate methods. In particular, at least in some areas of psychology, there is argument about the value of scientific versus qualitative, interpretive approaches. Qualitative methods are now more widely accepted within the discipline. Their possible value for investigations into the experience of chronic illness and disability is certainly worthy of consideration.

What are my views in this matter? What are my views now that I myself am a person with disabilities? In my pre-MS days as a psychologist I was in the position of the researcher. When I was teaching about a particular topic, I was usually commenting on research carried out by other people. Nevertheless, I was still, in a sense, identifying with those who were carrying out the research.

Now things are different in an important sense. I have become a member of a group *subject* to research. I have a kind of dual identity as researcher, but also as a respondent, a participant in the research. Has this had an influence in the way that I think about and evaluate the research process?

To some extent my acceptance of the value of qualitative research has increased. Now, as a participant in such research, I can say that I have found it a more enjoyable and engaging experience than being a respondent in scientific, quantitative research. Qualitative research provides an opportunity to comment on experience from the inside, so to speak. Of course, the researcher has his or her own research framework, which may be constraining to some extent, but there is usually a degree of open-endedness and flexibility involved. The personal encounter which is part of such research is likely to be positive and encouraging.

But, as is indicated by my earlier comments on the 'Loss of Self' research, qualitative research is also open to criticism. Firstly qualitative research, by its nature, involves a process of interpretation. So, is the 'right' interpretation being made? But, what *is* the correct interpretation in this context? Obviously, there are complex issues which cannot be explored in detail here.[13] The most important response is to say that the interpretations made need to be supported through a chain of evidence and argument that draw directly on the actual responses made by the participants in the research.

My new position as a member of a researched group means that I want to go a little further than this. At least some qualitative researchers now argue that research respondents should be seen as co-researchers.[14] As John Heron puts it, such research should be *with* people, not *on* them. At its strongest, such an approach would mean that those who are being subject to research would be involved in all stages of the research process. At the very least it should mean that interpretations made by the researchers are checked out with the respondents in the investigation.

An important issue in relation to all research is that of the extent to which the researchers are able to draw conclusions beyond the particular group of people they have actually investigated. This is the issue of generalisation – to what extent do the findings obtained apply to other people, beyond those actually investigated?

This is a particularly difficult problem in the context of qualitative research because samples are often small, and may not be fully representative of the wider population.[15] Some qualitative researchers would say that this kind of generalisation is not their objective. They are more concerned with finding how things are within a particular group, or with generalising on a theoretical, rather than statistical, basis. In that case the researchers need to avoid suggestions that their conclusions apply to people in general. One of my quarrels with Kathy Charmaz, at least in the article I have quoted from, is that she appears to be suggesting that her findings about 'loss of self' apply to *all* people who are chronically ill.

Thus, there are potential difficulties in the qualitative approach to research, but it is one that is undergoing rapid development. In particular, clearer criteria for evaluating good qualitative research are now emerging. As far as I'm concerned, my experience on both sides of the research divide leads me to think that qualitative research makes an important contribution to our better understanding of the experience of chronic illness and disability. I would very much agree with the position taken by Timothy Elliott and colleagues who write that,

> *To understand the cognitive mechanisms underlying optimal adjustment...it is imperative that we develop and use qualitative devices that are sensitive to the perceptions and beliefs through which people find meaning rather than despair following disability.*[16]

Sad Times...

I have mentioned that my father died – in February 2005, a week before his ninetieth birthday. He had been very fortunate, in many ways, in both his life and career. He saw the development of a new discipline – international politics – in a department often described as the 'home of the discipline'. He lectured there for 35 years and over that time saw a great expansion in size, and major development in its academic reputation. He ended his career as head of department and holder of the Wilson chair of international politics. He maintained his contact with the department into retirement as professor emeritus.

My mother was already ninety when my father died, but still in pretty good form. She was, for instance, still cycling the mile or so down a non-traffic, tree-lined avenue which took her to the edge of the Aberystwyth shopping area; she was also making bread, five pounds of flour at a time, more than once a week. I expected, hoped that she would be with us for a while longer, but sadly it was not to be.

My mother was diagnosed with cancer in the autumn of 2005, less than a year after Dad's death. Even at the age of ninety-one, she put up a valiant fight, deciding to undergo chemotherapy which gave her, and us, some extra time. She coped stoically in a way that I'm not sure that I could have done. But the end was inevitable and my mother died, at the age of ninety-two, on the 13th of October 2006, twenty months after my father.

I have found it harder to cope with my mother's death, I'm sure for a number of reasons. It was the second death within a relatively short period of time; now I had lost both parents. Mum was central to our family life, but a much more private person than my father. In many ways, on his death, we were boyed up by the very many supportive messages we received from his old friends, immediate ex-colleagues, the wider disciplinary community, and also extended obituary notices. Mum's funeral was a quieter, a more subdued occasion with family and immediate friends.

Also, Mum was ill for a longer period of time, and we had to witness her slow decline. There were some greater feelings of guilt on my part – I couldn't be in Aberystwyth all the time, but had feelings that I should have been there more. Probably, as one friend said, 'mothers are different' – the early close emotional relationship has an impact. Its disruption is more painful.

There were still some more positive times during this difficult period. When Pete and I were in Aberystwyth we were able to take Mum out in the 'baby bus'. At the end this was just for rides, but during most of the period Mum was able to come for short walks. She did enjoy these. Although I am pretty sure that my mother has never read any Buddhist literature, she was still able to enjoy the moment. She continued to be very appreciative of natural beauty.

The most important event over the summer of 2006 was that my sister Mair, her husband Rich and my niece Carys were able to come over from Boston. Carys, at 21, was a fully independent operator. She came over separately from her parents and with her boyfriend Andy, and one of her girlfriends, Sarah. The young people had first of all spent some time in London, and travelling out from there a little. Then they came down to Aberystwyth, which Carys knows well, and stayed for a bit over a week. Their visit overlapped with that of Mair and Rich.

I must admit to some concern over how my mother would cope with such an influx of lively and inevitably noisy young people. But she did cope and related well to the young people – she was meeting Andy and Sarah for the first time. As they were not staying in the same house, it helped that she was able to see them in small doses. It was a good and important time for all of us, and we were so fortunate that my mother was well enough to get enjoyment and great satisfaction from the visit.

Mum died at home as she had wished. Although one hears a lot that is negative, we really couldn't fault the care my mother received from the NHS. There were sometimes delays with ambulance lifts, but almost always there was a bed available when needed. Care received at home from the district nurse team over the last couple of months was really excellent. Of greatest importance was the care and love given by my sister. Ceri has lived at home with my parents for a number of years, so she was on the spot. But giving the kind of close personal care needed at this kind of time is not an easy thing to do. Ceri managed it wonderfully well.

Onward...

Life goes on. Now I have had MS for fifteen years. I think, on the whole, I am doing reasonably well. There are times of struggle and periods of melancholy. But there are also good times; there are many things to enjoy. There are opportunities which would not be there if I didn't have MS. At its simplest I can go out when the sun shines!

I have, of course, been very lucky. Not lucky to get MS, but I have been very fortunate in so many other ways. Unlike many people who become chronically ill and disabled I have not been under major financial pressure. Many people lose their previous income, and at the same time you soon realise when you are disabled that the things you need (wheelchairs etc.) are very expensive. I have also been hugely fortunate to have a supportive husband who was able to accept and adjust to my becoming ill.

I have also perhaps been fortunate in the way that my MS has developed. I haven't had the positive benefit of regular remissions but, on the other hand, I haven't had to cope with the uncertain ups and downs which are a part of the relapse remission form of MS. Also, so far, my progressive MS (if that is what it is) has taken a generally stable, steady course rather than one which has involved serious deterioration.

I count myself as someone who is moderately, rather than severely disabled. As I've recounted, even moderate disability can be quite restricting and exasperating. However, I know that it could have been much more so, and I am grateful for the many things that I can still do.

So how do I continue to occupy my days? The motivational 'web' still develops and expands, but perhaps also frays a little at some of its edges. I finished my Esperanto course, but have to admit that my study here is in abeyance at the moment – I may come back to it later. I have been reading a fair bit of history – although not in a very disciplined way. I may well get myself involved in a formal, probably Open University correspondence course at some time. As well as learning a bit of Esperanto I also learned that correspondence courses suit me quite well.

The most important new departure is that in September 2005 I joined Sandbach U3A. The University of the Third Age is a national organisation with independent 'branches' in many places throughout the country. Sandbach U3A had been founded a couple of years earlier – somehow without my noticing it! Each U3A is a kind of self help community of adult learners who are free of work commitments.

Members teach and learn with each other. There are no certificates awarded, or qualifications sought. Groups that focus on physical activity of some kind and those promoting artistic endeavours are as important as those which are more intellectual in character.

I really enjoy this shared learning situation, especially as fellow U3A members are usually enthusiastic and keen to participate and contribute. U3A for me, and many others, is an important source of companionship and friendship. It provides a structured situation in which it is possible to get-together with like-minded people on a regular basis.

Our links with Aberystwyth are still an important part of our lives. With my two sisters I now own what was my parents' house. My sister, Ceri, continues to live there. Pete and I visit frequently. We take the opportunity to meet up with our friends who live there.

Presently, life is certainly busy and enjoyable. I know now that there will be difficulties and challenges but I do have some appreciation of their nature. I also know that life could turn more uncertain at any point. I need to ensure that I do not dwell on this. Life is an uncertain business for everybody. I hope that I will be able to keep living in a reasonably positive kind of way – writing this book has helped towards this.

> *...telling the stories of our lives, making sense of what otherwise seems chaotic, distilling and discovering a trajectory in our lives, and viewing our lives with a sense of agency rather than victimhood are all powerfully positive.*[17]

Now, at the end of 2008, there has been another change, a positive one, and nothing to do with MS. Pete has retired from his lecturing job. There will be a different kind of life for us both – more time and new opportunities.

Notes and References

1. These two articles are Bury, M. (1982). Chronic illness as biographical disruption. *Sociology of Health and Illness*, 4, 167-82. and Williams, G. H. (1984). The genesis of chronic illness: narrative reconstruction. *Sociology of Health and Illness*, 6, 174-200.

2. Charmaz, K. (1983). Loss of self: a fundamental form of suffering in the chronically ill. *Sociology of Health and Illness*, 5, 2, 168-195. The quoted comments are from pages 168-169.

3. These criticisms are developed in Cuthbert, K (1999). Experience of self in the context of chronic illness. *Health Psychology Update*, 36, 11-15.

4. Despite his very severe disability Christopher Reeve clearly asserted his continuing sense of self and identity. Reeve, C. (1998). *Still Me*. London: Century.

5. This article is Albrecht, G.L. and Devlieger, P.J. (1998). The disability paradox: high quality of life against all odds. *Social Science & Medicine* 48, 977-988

6. Reynolds, F., & Prior, S. (2003). Sticking jewels in your life: Exploring women's strategies for negotiating an acceptable quality of life with multiple sclerosis. *Qualitative Health Research*, 13, 9, 1225-1251.

7. Seymour Epstein's ideas were introduced in the second chapter of this book.

8. The idea of self-narrative was introduced in Chapter two of this book. A good introductory commentary on this narrative approach in the context of chronic illness is provided in Crossley, M. L. (2000). *Introducing Narrative Psychology: Self, trauma and the construction of meaning*. Buckingham: Open University Press.

9. Two key figures in the emergence of positive psychology are Martin Seligman and Mihaly Csikszentmihalyi. They wrote the lead introductory article for that special edition of the American Psychologist. Seligman, M., & Csikszentmihalyi, M. (2000). Positive psychology: an introduction. *American Psychologist*, 55, 5-14.

10. Snyder, C.R. & Lopez, S.J. (Eds) (2002). *Handbook of Positive Psychology*. New York: Oxford University Press.

11. Boniwell, I. (2006). *Positive Psychology in a Nutshell*. London: PWBC.

12. Elliot, T. R., Kurylo, M., & Rivera, P. (2002). Positive growth following acquired physical disability. in C. R. Snyder & S. J. Lopez (Eds), *Handbook of Positive Psychology*, pp. 687-699. New York: Oxford University Press. The quotation is from p.688.

13. These issues are, of course, being explored in a variety of current journals and books. One such, which reviews qualitative approaches in the context of health psychology, is Murray, M.' & Chamberlin, K. (1999) (Eds). *Qualitative Health Psychology: Theories and methods*. London: Sage Publications.

14. This is a position which has been taken for quite some time by John Rowan, Peter Reason and John Heron. An early contribution, for example, was by Peter Reason in a volume co-edited with John Rowan: Reason, P. (1981). An exploration of the dialectics of two-person relationships. in P.Reason, & J. Rowan, (Eds) *Human Inquiry: A sourcebook of New Paradigm Research*, Chichester: John Wiley. A more recent contribution is Reason, P. & Heron, J. (1995) Co-operative Inquiry. in J. A. Smith, Harre, R., & Van Langenhove, L. (Eds.), *Rethinking Methods in Psychology*, London: Sage Publications.

15. There is increasing examination of this issue. a good discussion of generalisation in the context of qualitative research is provided, for example, in Schofield, J. W. (1993). Increasing the Generalizability of Qualitative Research. in M. Hammersley (Ed). *Social Research: Philosophy, politics and practice*, London: Sage.

16. Elliot et al (2002). The quotation is from p.695 in the article Positive growth following acquired physical disability, cited above.

17. Seligman, M. E. P. (2002). Positive psychology, positive prevention and positive therapy. in C. R. Snyder & S. J. Lopez (Eds), *Handbook of Positive Psychology*, pp. 3-9 New York: Oxford University Press. The quotation is taken from p. 7.

Index